FATAL
DECEPTION

FATAL
DECEPTION

THE UNTOLD STORY OF ASBESTOS

WHY IT IS STILL LEGAL AND STILL KILLING US

MICHAEL BOWKER

RODALE

© 2003 by Michael Bowker

Photographs © by EyeWire/Getty Images (cover); Michael Brown Productions (aerial view of smoke coming out of mill); *The Western News* (Gov. Martz); CinemaPhoto/CORBIS (Steve McQueen); Reuters NewMedia Inc./CORBIS (Elmo Zumwalt, WTC site); Mark M. Lawrence/CORBIS (N.Y. firefighter)

Printed in the United States of America

Rodale Inc. makes every effort to use acid-free ∞, recycled paper ♲ .

Cover Designer: Joanna Williams
Interior photographs courtesy of Katherine Jorgensen (two boys playing); Susan Vento and the Mesothelioma Applied Research Foundation (Bruce Vento); the Runyan Collection at the Heritage Museum in Libby, MT (Vermiculite Mountain, baseball field); the Environmental Protection Agency ("EPA crews remove asbestos-contaminated soils . . . ," EPA trucks, running track, Grace's screening plant, Rainy Creek Road); and Michael Bowker

Library of Congress Cataloging-in-Publication Data

Bowker, Michael, date.
    Fatal deception : the untold story of asbestos : why it is still legal and still killing us / Michael Bowker.
        p. ; cm.
    ISBN 1–57954–684–6 hardcover
    1. Asbestos—Health aspects.   2. Asbestos—Environmental aspects.   I. Title.
    [DNLM: 1. Asbestos—adverse effects—Popular Works.   2. Environmental Exposure—Popular Works.   3. Industry—Popular Works.   4. Public Policy—Popular Works.   WA 754 B786f   2003]
    RA1231.A8 B69   2003
    363.17'91—dc21
                                                             2002152241

Distributed to the book trade by St. Martin's Press

2   4   6   8   10   9   7   5   3   1   hardcover

Visit us on the Web at www.rodalestore.com, or call us toll-free at (800) 848-4735.

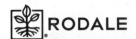

WE **INSPIRE** AND **ENABLE** PEOPLE TO IMPROVE
THEIR LIVES AND THE WORLD AROUND THEM

To my mother, Ellyn Larsen,
whose unshakable belief in happy endings
is still the best part of me.

"When you can't breathe, nothing else matters."
—The American Lung Association

ACKNOWLEDGMENTS

The enthusiastic and discerning research conducted by Sharon Bowker, my beautiful and talented sister, greatly enriched this book. I also want to thank Heide Lange, my agent, who made it all happen; Chris Potash for his fine editorial hand; Joanna Williams for her cover design; and especially Stephanie Tade and Rodale for believing in this project from the beginning. Many thanks, also, to the dozens of attorneys, doctors, scientists, and international researchers, such as Dr. Alan Whitehouse in Spokane; Dr. Aubrey Miller in Denver; and Laurie Kazan-Allen in London, who lent me their valuable time and expertise; to Doug Eikermann, my friend since the beginning of time, who as an author has experienced the joy and anguish of creation; Jennifer Kushnier for her research assistance; and to the guys in EPA's Region 8, whose plan of attack should be emulated by emergency response teams everywhere.

Like every writer working on the story of asbestos, I owe a debt of gratitude to the two men whose work was seminal in exposing the misdeeds of the industry, Paul Brodeur and Barry Castleman. Their voices should have been heeded long ago.

My special thanks to the residents of Libby, Montana, and those asbestos victims in the United States and around the world who shared their personal stories with me. Their astonishing courage provided more inspiration than any writer could use in a lifetime.

Finally, huge hugs to Jody, Kristine, and Michele, whose support and energy were endless and essential.

CONTENTS

PREFACE

The challenge of any story is the telling. That was especially true in the creation of this book because the story of asbestos is as braided and complex as the fiber itself. There are major financial, medical, political, legal, and, most of all, personal storylines, and each plays a major role. Structuring the book was a daunting task because detailing each of these elements could easily fill volumes. Moreover, during the research, unexpected and important tributaries appeared at every turn, complicating and enriching the story.

One of these is the mystifying scandal involving the EPA that may have caused many of the thirty thousand people in lower Manhattan to be exposed to high levels of deadly asbestos fibers from the World Trade Center collapse. Another is the fact that asbestos remains at the heart of a multibillion-dollar legal war that has dozens of major American companies on the brink of financial disaster.

The biggest challenge was how to fit all of these into one book. Certainly, the national and international scope of the problem formed a major thread, but so too did the ongoing and heartbreaking personal stories of the people in Libby, Montana, the site of the largest environmental disaster in U.S. history. Libby was polluted with deadly asbestos fibers for more than sixty years, until recently, when a handful of courageous residents stood up and fought for their town and families. One of these heroes was Robert Wilkins, who died of asbestos-related causes on November 10, 2002, and in whose memory this book is written.

The events in Libby are crucial to the story because they explode several myths about asbestos, including the misconception that asbestos poisoning is strictly occupational in nature. More than fourteen hundred people in Libby have been stricken, and only a few were miners. The medical studies in Libby are greatly expanding our understanding of asbestos-related diseases, and the EPA has also discovered new ways in which asbestos fibers can invade and hide in our homes.

To understand the full threat of asbestos, I felt it was important to plait both of these stories into one. In large part, the national story runs on a parallel course to Libby's, but there are a few major intersections—particularly the World Trade Center, which included tons of deadly asbestos from the Libby mine. The two stories are told in alternating chapters in chronological form, more or less.

Of the more than one hundred interviews that took place during the research for this book, none were more inspiring or more difficult than the ones I did with asbestos victims in Libby and elsewhere around the country. I found that their personal courage mirrored that which we all saw displayed by the victims of the 9/11 tragedy. The difference is that the hundreds of thousands of asbestos victims remain this nation's darkest secret. This book is dedicated to them. May it shed a light.

Michael Bowker
Placerville, California
Autumn, 2002

FATAL
DECEPTION

1

SERPENT IN THE ROCK

Tucked into a wild, verdant valley in the northwestern part of Montana, surrounded by a deep wilderness that extends well beyond the Canadian border ninety miles to the north, lies the town of Libby. John Steinbeck once called Montana "A Love Affair," and so it is with Libby. Those who love the solitude, natural beauty, and physical independence that the town offers are compelled to live here, even though jobs often are scarce.

The twelve thousand or so folks who live around Libby are friendly, open, and trusting, for the most part. They are aware of their backwater status and are quick to make self-deprecating jokes about it. But, the truth is, they love Libby and wouldn't live anywhere else.

The bucolic, pine-rimmed valley, the jade-colored Kootenai River, and the snowcapped Cabinet Mountains that arc some seven thousand feet above the town combine to make Libby an idyllic village of postcard views. Life is simple and quiet here. Everyone knows one another. The crime rate is low. Bar fights and moose-poaching reports take up most of the police ledger, and it has been that way for more than a hundred years.

That's why the last thing anyone expected was that Libby would suddenly become Ground Zero for the most lethal environmental poisoning in U.S. history. No one could have predicted that this small American town was about to become the center of a medical, legal, and political storm over asbestos that would make headlines around the world. And no one could have imagined that hundreds and perhaps thousands of people would ultimately die in Libby from tiny fibers no one could see. A snake had entered Paradise, and nobody saw it coming.

Asbestos is the general term for a number of naturally occurring fibrous forms of several mineral silicates. These grow in chainlike crystal structures of billions of microscopic fibers that are so light they can float in the air for hours or even days. The fibers are so pliable they can be woven into cloth.

Because it is literally a rock, asbestos is waterproof, fireproof, and corrosion-proof. Manufacturers quickly found that this "magic mineral" had hundreds of applications in buildings, homes, appliances, automobiles, and in a variety of common products from ironing board pads and cigarette filters to hair dryers and children's clothing.

Besides its insulating and fireproofing properties, asbestos has the tensile strength of piano wire, making it perfect for use as a binding agent in thousands of building products such as cement, tile, mastics, and vinyl wall and floor coverings. More than thirty-three million tons of it have been incorporated in buildings, vehicles, and products in the United States, greatly boosting the fortunes of dozens of great American companies such as Johns Manville, Raybestos-Manhattan, Owens Corning, and W. R. Grace. Asbestos was indeed a "miracle mineral" when it came to profit margins.

The problem with asbestos is the fibers. They break off at the slightest provocation. Needle-sharp and shaped like spears, they can be inhaled by the thousands with each breath. Some physicians believe even one of the fibers, lodged in the wrong place, can eventually kill a person. While many of the fibers find their way safely out of the body, others inevitably embed themselves in soft tissue and cannot be removed. They most often lodge in the lungs and lining of the abdomen but have been found in nearly every major organ of the human body, including the brain and the heart.

Asbestos exposure is related to increased levels of several types of cancer, especially of the lungs and stomach. Asbestos is the sole cause of mesothelioma (*mees-o-thee-lee-o-na*), a virulent and fatal cancer that doctors say is more physically painful and psychologically devastating than AIDS. It also causes asbestosis, a serious, progressive, and potentially fatal disease that eventually kills its victims by cutting off their oxygen supply. Asbestosis can lie dormant and then suddenly "flower," causing death in a relatively short time; its victims are said to have ticking time bombs inside their chests.

"Asbestos-related diseases can cause pain, shortness of breath, inability to eat, and heart problems," said Dr. Harvey Pass, head of thoracic oncology at the Barbara Ann Karmanos Cancer Institute in Detroit. "If you can't eat or breathe and your heart doesn't work very well and you're having pain during this, you tend to wither away and suffer tremendously—that's pretty awful. Yet, as aware as our society is about most diseases, these still go unnoticed."

The failure of other organs due to the stress of diminished oxygen, and the overall lack of understanding in America of asbestos-related diseases, are reasons experts feel the number of asbestos victims has been vastly underestimated. "We'll never know how many people whose death certificates indicate the cause of death to be heart attacks, lung disease, kidney failure, or some other problem, who actually died of asbestos-related diseases," said Dr. Aubrey Miller, an asbestos expert with the U.S. Public Health Service. "But the number has to be very high."

In northwestern Montana, that number has been growing

steadily for decades. The poison that crept so quietly into Libby has been at work for generations, much as it has been throughout the rest of America. It would have continued to reap its terrible harvest in secret—and the serious dangers posed by asbestos swept under the rug completely—if it hadn't been for a few troublemakers in Libby who wouldn't shut up.

Leaning back in an easy chair in his small apartment overlooking Libby's Little League ballpark, Bob Wilkins doesn't look much like a troublemaker. His eyes are still vibrant and full of fire, but his skin is tight and has taken on a gray pallor. A prideful, handsome man, Wilkins is a former chief of police who once kept the peace in the boisterous, Wild West town of Wolf Point, Montana. It was a physical job, dealing with drunks and rowdies and cowboys whooping it up on weekends. You have a feeling he was up to the task. He still has the firm jawline and physical bearing of a man who could take care of himself in a scrap. He used to keep in shape hiking the mountains with his children and running five miles a day. He'll tell you that with obvious pride. Today, he has trouble walking down the single flight of stairs to his car. Asbestosis has eaten away 70 percent of his lungs.

"I first came to Libby in 1966," he said, his words interrupted by a constant cough. "The job I was promised at the mine paid more than I was making in Wolf Point, and I loved the area. It was an open pit mine so we would be working outside. It sounded good to me." Wilkins's wife, Louise, and their five children were excited and relieved by the move. Louise felt that working for a big corporation like W. R. Grace, which owned the mine, was a much safer job than keeping the peace in Wolf Point.

Wilkins worked at the screening plant that perched on the

banks of the Kootenai (*Coot-nee*) River. The ore was trucked down from the mountain, and once it was screened, sized, and graded, Wilkins was in charge of loading it into the Burlington Northern railcars and sending it to destinations around the world. As he worked, bald eagles and osprey wheeled above and fished in the Kootenai, and bighorn sheep and elk roamed the forests and cliffs around him. "I thought I had the best job on earth," he said.

Today, he knows differently. Interlaced with the ore was a mineral called tremolite, one of the most lethal forms of asbestos. Asbestos fibers were released into the atmosphere by the millions in nearly every step of the mining process. The screening plant was dusty all the time. Wilkins was covered with it nearly every day. The company kept the dangers of the tremolite secret from the miners and the town until hundreds of people in Libby had died and more than fourteen hundred others were diagnosed with asbestos-related diseases.

Wilkins's favorite T-shirt, the one he wears around Libby on the good days when he can get out, reads: LOCAL 361 GAVE ME A WATCH, W. R. GRACE GAVE ME ASBESTOS.

The sentiments do not amuse those who represent W. R. Grace, the multibillion-dollar chemical and oil conglomerate based in Columbia, Maryland.

"The Grace people give me hell about it—they say I'm stirring up trouble," Wilkins said. "But I told them, after all the pain you've caused this town, you're lucky that's all I'm doing."

As Wilkins talked, his eyes were constantly moving. They seemed alternately bewildered, angry, and questioning. "See that over there," Wilkins said, pointing to an ugly, rusting, corrugated iron building rising above the baseball dugout. "We called it the popping plant. It was part of the mine operation. That's where they took the ore to heat it. There used to be four Little League baseball diamonds surrounding it. Dust would be flying out of the popping plant all the time, covering those ball fields. The guys who ran the mine told us not to worry, that it was just a nuisance dust."

Wilkins closed his eyes and for a moment it seemed as though he had gone to sleep. When he opened them again, it was apparent he was crying. "Had we known, none of us would have ever worked there," he said softly. "We didn't know the dust was killing all those women and children."

Les Skramstad remembers the day in 1959 when he was told to bring one of the company pickup trucks to one of the high levels of the huge, bulldozed, terraced area of the mine. "We backed the truck up to a huge pile of stuff and loaded it with our hands," Skramstad said. "It was pure asbestos. They were experimenting with it. We had to bring it down to the plant and clean it. I remember the boss—this was before W. R. Grace bought the mine in 1963—came over to us and said, 'We have so much asbestos up here we have to find a market for it. If we do, we'll be in business forever. There ain't no limit to this stuff. It's all over this mountain.'"

Skramstad, a trim, rugged-looking man who looks like he just walked out of central casting for a cowboy movie, is sitting in a Libby restaurant with his wife, Norita. They are both Libby troublemakers. They got that way after they and three of their five children were diagnosed with asbestos-caused diseases.

"I only worked at that mine for two and a half years," Skramstad said. "But they had us down on our hands and knees sorting through the asbestos. We built a screen-and-shaker so we could separate out the rocks. They wanted the asbestos to be pure. They were trying to see if they could manufacture a product out of it. All the material was wet because there were natural springs all over the mountain. We had to dry it with electric heaters. By the time we were done, we'd go home covered with asbestos dust. The kids would hug me and get it all over themselves. Norita would wash my clothes and she'd get contaminated. We had no idea it was lethal. No one at the mine ever said a word."

Skramstad quit his job at the mine in 1961, but by then it was too late. "Never in my wildest dreams did I ever think that I was doing anything to hurt my family," he said, his voice suddenly breaking. "That's what makes me the maddest. They gave me a job that had fatal consequences and knowingly let me take that death home to my wife and kids. You tell me, what kind of people could do that?"

At the W. R. Grace headquarters in 1963, the opportunity to buy the Libby mine that yielded the strange and rare ore called vermiculite was too good to pass up. J. Peter Grace, the company's young, ambitious president and CEO, was convinced that purchasing the mine would yield a new product that could penetrate nearly unlimited untapped markets.

Vermiculite, which in its raw form is a shiny, blackish rock with the layered consistency of shale, has one amazing characteristic: When heated, the water trapped inside its layers turns to steam and "pops" the vermiculite, much like a kernel of popcorn. The vermiculite suddenly expands to about seventeen times its original size, turns a gold color, and gains an airy consistency. In its expanded form, vermiculite is used in insulation, animal feed, potting soil, gypsum plaster, fertilizer, brake pads, fireproof safes, paints, fireplaces, and a host of other products.

The vermiculite deposit, which sits on the top of a low mountain about six miles north of Libby, is one of the largest ever found in the world. It covers more than twelve hundred acres and extends from the surface to dozens of feet underground. Mining and processing the ore was a relatively simple but extremely dusty process.

For W. R. Grace, one of the world's largest manufacturers of specialty chemicals, the purchase of the mine proved to be a highly profitable move. With help of a national advertising campaign that starred comedian Danny Kaye and others, the demand for vermiculite skyrocketed. Orders came from all over the United States, Japan, France, England, Canada, and several other countries. Before long, Grace was processing thousands of tons per day.

There was only one problem. Since 1940, Montana state health officials had been concerned about the dust emissions at the mine. In 1962, a year before W. R. Grace bought the mine, the state determined that the dust contained high levels of tremolite asbestos that was dangerous to human health.

By 1963, however, Peter Grace was emerging as one of the most powerful and well-connected corporate figures in America. A serious and determined man, Grace had taken over the helm of W. R. Grace in 1945, when he was only thirty-two years old. The company was founded in 1854 by his grandfather, William Russell Grace, who also initiated the family's entrée into the political world when he served two terms as the mayor of New York City. As mayor, he accepted the Statue of Liberty from the French in 1885. He also built a steamship line that created service from New York to South America, where the company had several business operations. William Grace was a tough, swashbuckling corporate giant of the ilk of John Rockefeller and J. P. Morgan.

Grandson Peter was born to power, wealth, and privilege. Like his grandfather, he was a driven man. Not only did he pursue his dream of expanding the Grace corporate empire, he was extremely active in politics and governmental operations at a high level. Polished, urbane, and extremely conservative, he enjoyed close relationships with presidents, popes, CIA directors, and a multitude of other highly placed politicians. He served as the head of the Commerce Department Committee on the Alliance for Progress under President John Kennedy and would play a high-profile role in the Reagan administration. He also maintained a close relationship with the Bush family, which would ultimately yield two American presidents.

By 1963, Peter Grace had already expanded the company's operations to New Zealand, Japan, France, Germany, Italy, and Australia. He was confident that he could deal with a few backwoods Montana health officials.

Besides Wilkins and Skramstad, people like Bob Dedrick, who grew up in a house next to the popping plant, and Jim Racicot, the cousin of a former Montana governor, helped bring the story to the front pages. Dedrick, a gentle man who for forty straight years took out a moose hunting permit—but who could never talk himself into shooting one—took dead aim at the W. R. Grace company after his cousin died of mesothelioma and his uncle of asbestosis. Dedrick, his wife, and his brother have since been diagnosed with asbestos-caused diseases.

Racicot, a fun-loving, amiable man who often answers his phone "GOOD MORNING, MONNNNTANA!" has, along with his twin brother, younger brother, and sister, been diagnosed with asbestosis. Although Racicot's father and stepfather also died of the poison dust from the mine, he felt his cousin, Marc Racicot, nominated by George W. Bush and elected in January 2002 to head the Republican National Committee, did not do enough to help the people of Libby during his term as governor of Montana during the 1990s. "It has caused a bit of a rift in the family," Racicot said.

Both Dedrick and Jim Racicot played key roles in exposing the Libby situation, as did a blond, boisterous, intelligent, and angry grandmother of eleven named Gayla Benefield. Benefield, perhaps the most unlikely troublemaker of all, was for most of her life content to take care of her family and their log home along a beautiful bend of the Kootenai River. Being in the public spotlight had always made her uncomfortable. That was before she lost her mother and father to the mine dust, and before she, her husband, one of her daughters, and thirty-four other members of her extended family were diagnosed with potentially fatal lung abnormalities.

"Troublemaker?" repeated Benefield. "Oh yes, I plan to make as much trouble as I can for W. R. Grace before I die."

Motivated by what she calls a case of "corporate murder," Benefield has emerged as a tough-talking media magnet who has told her story to national magazines and television news stations throughout the country. She can still remember the day, September 17, 1954, on her eleventh birthday, when her father, Perley Vatland, came to her with wonderful news. Perley had just been offered a job at the vermiculite mine. It was huge news because Perley was unemployed, and jobs at the mine were hard to get. Everyone in town wanted to work there. The jobs paid well, and besides, the company offered good health benefits.

At the time the job seemed to be a dream come true to Perley and his wife, Margaret. Norwegian immigrants, they had moved to Libby in 1946 after giving up on a hardscrabble farm in North Dakota. Perley and Margaret came to Montana in search of a better life for their children.

"My dad gave me a hug that day and told me it was my birthday present," Gayla said with a small laugh. "It always seemed special to me. Not too many kids get a job for their birthday."

An ecstatic Perley told the family, "This is the job of a lifetime."

All Gayla knew was that the entire family was happy. "It was like, 'Dad's got a job, now everything is going to be all right,'" she said.

As the new man at the mine, Perley's first job was working as a sweeper in the dry mill. Each day after work he arrived home covered in a thick white dust. Sometimes Margaret would brush him off with a broom outside in the yard. Otherwise, Gayla remembered, he would walk directly into the house and get his cup of coffee that Margaret always had ready for him. Margaret washed his dusty clothes twice a week.

The dust at the mine was ubiquitous, but the men tolerated it with a shrug. "No worse than farm dust," they were told. It seemed a small price to pay for a steady job in Libby that offered a twenty-year retirement pension.

Ten years later, the price had escalated. Perley had come down with a series of lung ailments he didn't seem to be able to shake. Once robust and able to work long hours, his health broke down, and he suffered greatly over the next decade. He was stunned that the managers at W. R. Grace didn't seem to care. "He felt they turned their backs on him after he had worked so hard for them," Gayla said.

Perley died five days before he would have made his twenty-year pension. His last months were filled with suffering. He was unable to breathe much of the time, and his chest felt like it was on fire. After he died, the company declined to pay his full pension to the family. No one from W. R. Grace called the family with condolences or sent flowers or even a card.

"Mom received thirty-seven dollars a month from the company," Gayla said. "That's what Dad's life was worth."

Gayla's mother was fifty-four years old when she lost her husband. She had never worked outside the home, but she learned to sell Avon products and managed to just make ends meet. But in

1978, Margaret, too, began to feel sick. Her strength slowly diminished, as did her lung capacity. The doctors diagnosed pneumonia and other respiratory diseases, but in 1986 she was finally diagnosed with asbestosis. Her disease was slow acting but relentless. After spending her final two years in constant pain and agony, Margaret died in 1996. She died knowing it was the dust on Perley's clothes that had killed her. A happy, gentle woman for most of her life, she spent her last days bitter and angry.

Just before her death, Margaret had asked Gayla to move to her bedside. "Gayla, I want you to promise me one thing," her mother whispered in a rasping voice. "I want you to promise me you will get them—you'll get the bastards who did this to me."

Gayla took only a moment to answer. "I will," she said. "Oh, I will."

2

A PLAGUE OF EPIC
PROPORTIONS

Most Americans mistakenly believe that asbestos was permanently banned in the United States years ago. It wasn't. Although medical evidence long ago proved conclusively that asbestos is lethal, it remains a legal ingredient in more than three thousand products nationwide, including paint, toasters, ovens, dishwashers, fireplaces, pipes and pipe insulation, automobile brake shoes, chalkboards, and even shotgun shells.

"People who think that asbestos is yesterday's problem are dead wrong," said Chris Weis, an EPA asbestos coordinator in Denver. "It's shocking to me that hundreds of thousands of people are dying of asbestos-related disease across this country but most people don't know a thing about it. Maybe they have heard about asbestos for so many years they think it is no longer a danger. But it is causing a plague of epic proportions. People need to understand that."

Although few consumers were aware of it, more than 250,000 tons of asbestos were imported and used in American products between 1991 and 2001, according to the United States Geological Survey. Not only that, but millions of tons of asbestos remain in residential and commercial buildings across America. The occupants, as well as electricians, plumbers, and others who maintain the buildings, may be subjected to dangerous levels of asbestos every day.

Because the story of the asbestos has not yet fully penetrated the consciousness of most Americans, it continues to kill with silent, horrifying efficiency. By the year 2030, asbestos is expected to be listed as the official cause of death of about five hundred thousand Americans. Due to the underreporting of asbestos-related diseases, however, many medical experts believe that the true death toll from asbestos will be four to ten times that many people in the United States, and far more worldwide.

The terrible events of September 11, 2001, brought asbestos back into the news as New Yorkers expressed well-founded fears regarding the contamination of lower Manhattan after the collapse of the World Trade Center. The WTC buildings contained hundreds of tons of asbestos. This included a fireproofing spray used on at least forty floors of the North Tower that was made from the asbestos-contaminated vermiculite from the Libby mine. Shortly after the WTC collapsed, higher asbestos levels were being found in the dust and soils in parts of lower Manhattan than were found in Libby.

The situation in New York remains serious, yet it is just the tip of the iceberg. Asbestos has been killing for years. One of its best-known victims was actor Steve McQueen, who played the cool good guy in movies like *Bullitt*, *The Getaway*, and *The Sand Pebbles*. McQueen was exposed to fibers as a young man when he took a job disassembling old, asbestos-laced ships. (Workers who built ships for the United States Navy in World War II suffered nearly the same mortality rate as the sailors who saw combat on those ships.) Like thousands of other victims of mesothelioma, McQueen was told there was no cure when he was diagnosed in 1979. He underwent an excruciating three-month experiment involving a treatment with laetrile, megadoses of vitamins, and other experimental medicines. As the cancer grew worse, he desperately tried a painful, radical surgery in Mexico because there was no treatment of any kind available in the United States.

Like the characters he portrayed, McQueen was a tough and valiant fighter, but there have been no known survivors of mesothelioma, a particularly potent and painful cancer. McQueen lost his battle with it in 1980. He was fifty years old. Today, mesothelioma patients face exactly the same fate because there have been no advancements in treatment options since McQueen was diagnosed, twenty-four years ago.

Asbestos is not a threat of the past. It is a present and future killer. Although caution labels are required by the Occupational Safety and Health Administration (OSHA) on raw asbestos materials in the workplace, there is virtually no labeling required on consumer products. Moreover, there is little monitoring done of the manufacture and use of asbestos-containing products, except when a worker complaint is filed. Government regulators rely almost entirely on industry data, despite the fact that the industry historically has been uncooperative. "Their strategy has always been to fight us tooth and nail," said Cindy Fraleigh, an attorney adviser for the EPA in Washington, D.C. "But we still rely on their data."

The U.S. government's approach to asbestos is paradoxical to the point of absurdity. The EPA, OSHA, and other federal and state regulatory agencies each have their own rules regarding the levels of asbestos fibers that are allowable and considered safe in homes and in the workplace. At the same time, the EPA's Web site states: "There is no known safe exposure level for asbestos."

That glaring contradiction, and the U.S. government's staunch seventy-year support of the asbestos industry, underscores one of the most deadly, ongoing events in American history. Steeped in secrecy, the story of asbestos is a revelation of immense corporate, po-

litical, and legal malfeasance. It is a story of profiteers who knowingly exposed unsuspecting workers and consumers to a sure and
painful death. Asbestos has already killed many times more Americans than did the war in Vietnam, and the human suffering continues to this day.

Journals from medical, insurance, and trade associations have
warned of the dangers of asbestos since the early 1900s. In its October 1935 issue, the *Eastern Underwriter* published reports on the
"alarming increase of asbestos cases" in the United States, and in
1934, the Aetna insurance company published the *Attorney's Text-
book of Medicine*, which included a chapter devoted solely to the
dangers of occupational asbestos exposure. It included a detailed
discussion of asbestosis, which it stated was "incurable and usually
results in total permanent disability followed by death."

Scores of other articles and reports were published on the dangers of asbestos in those early years, yet few workers or consumers
were ever told the full extent of the problem; indeed, the information was carefully hidden from them.

The medical costs of treating asbestos cancer victims in America are
projected to reach $500 billion within twenty-five years—and that
does not include tens and perhaps hundreds of billions of dollars
more for people who develop asbestosis, according to Barry
Castleman, an international expert on asbestos and author of *Asbestos: Medical and Legal Aspects* (Aspen Law and Business, 1996).
Wages lost by workers felled by asbestos-related diseases during that
time are expected to top $325 billion.

More than one hundred million Americans have already been
exposed to asbestos either on the job or at home, according to reports from the American Academy of Actuaries, an association of
insurance specialists. Especially at risk today are hundreds of thou-

sands of professional and do-it-yourself home remodelers who are being exposed to potentially dangerous levels of fibers as they tear out the asbestos-containing shingles, glues, plasters, paints, caulking, putty, floor and pipe coverings, siding, and insulation from older homes. Mechanics, too, are suffering high rates of asbestos-related diseases because many replacement brake shoes and clutches contain toxic levels of asbestos. Simply opening a box of asbestos brake shoes can release a dangerous number of fibers into the air.

The asbestos industry has sold America the concept that asbestos is safe as long as it remains sealed in place—as in cements and tiles—but nearly all asbestos products, as they age, become *friable*, a state where fibers can easily flake off into the atmosphere. Unlike most organic materials, which turn into dust particles when crushed or broken, asbestos breaks up into fine fibers that linger in the air. Even new asbestos roof tiles have been found to shed fibers when it rains, according to the London Hazards Centre.

The EPA estimated in the mid-1980s that about 20 percent of all public buildings in the United States contained some type of asbestos-containing friable material. That represents at least 733,000 buildings, including schools, hospitals, libraries, and public office buildings. In New York City alone, more than two-thirds of the existing buildings are believed to contain high levels of asbestos, and no one is sure how much of it is friable. The dangers this causes are twofold. First, those inside the buildings are potentially being exposed; millions of the microscopic fibers can become airborne without being seen.

The second danger comes from the fact that although asbestos abatement in buildings and homes can be done relatively safely, it is often done incorrectly. Studies in nine central Texas cities in the late 1990s showed that nearly 90 percent of the asbestos-removal projects undertaken by private companies grossly violated state and federal safety laws. Innovative Texas state laws have since curbed most of the abuses, but this type of widespread violation is likely to be occurring nationwide. Workers are often not fully trained, many do not have the proper equipment, and occupational monitoring is poor. Done incorrectly, asbestos removals can expose not only the workers to the fibers but also those who occupy the buildings after the job is finished.

A mélange of facts and actions have allowed asbestos to remain this nation's dark secret. The most obvious cause is the fact that for decades the asbestos industry successfully covered up the devastating effects of its product. Medical studies that showed high rates of sickness among workers were quashed, and company executives systematically failed to provide adequate information about the dangers of asbestos to their employees and consumers.

Secondly, until recently, the media never "got" the asbestos story. Reporters completely dropped the ball by failing to follow closely the EPA's attempt to outright ban asbestos in the United States. In 1989, the EPA had determined that no level of asbestos was safe and passed a phaseout program that would have banned asbestos entirely by 1996. The ban was challenged in court by the United States and Canadian asbestos industries and was overturned on a technicality by the 5th Circuit Court of Appeals in 1991. Rather than appeal the decision, or correct the technicality, President George Bush Sr. ordered the EPA to let the ban die, effectively legalizing asbestos use again in the United States. Confusion over the issue left the vast majority of Americans believing the ban was still in place.

A third factor is the socioeconomic and psychological makeup of the victims. Most were hardworking immigrants from Europe and Asia, grateful to have a job in this country. (Following that pattern, many of today's undertrained asbestcs abatement workers are Mexican immigrants.) The combination of their often unquestionable loyalty to the company and their fear cf being fired made them an exploitable workforce.

The wild card—and perhaps the most important ingredient in this witches' brew of concealment—is the fact that illness from asbestos exposure usually takes from ten to fifty years to manifest itself in serious symptoms. Had workers and consumers suffered symptoms immediately after exposure, concealment would not have been possible. But they couldn't see, taste, or touch the fibers they breathed in, nor could they feel the tiny spears penetrating the soft tissue of their lungs. There were no warning signals that the "nuisance dust," as it was called by the industry, was lethal. The miners, millers, and manufacturing workers would learn too late that it was deadly not only to them but also often to their families who were exposed to the asbestos dust they carried home on their work clothes.

This prolonged time lag from exposure to symptoms enabled the asbestos industry to continue to deny that asbestos was harmful. Years later, when workers and consumers became sick, industry officials blamed it on a host of other factors such as tobacco use or past operational practices.

Asbestos-related diseases have virtually been ignored by the government, and little federal money has been spent on research. The reason for this is deeply entangled in the corporate, legal, and political web of deceit and duplicity that has surrounded asbestos since the 1930s. An explosive story of greed, conspiracies, and ghastly moral choices, it seems like something out of the combined imaginations of Stephen King, Ayn Rand, and John Grisham.

From Franklin Roosevelt to Ronald Reagan and George Bush Sr., the asbestos industry's tentacles have reached the highest echelons of political power. The industry's footprints, via the Oval Office, are all over the backs of the regulatory agencies that repeatedly failed to protect workers and consumers. For example, when President Reagan organized a group to look into cutting governmental expenditures, in part by curbing the "overzealous" nature of regulatory government, he named his close friend Peter Grace to head what was to become known as the Grace Commission. Not surprisingly, governmental efforts to curb asbestos use subsequently withered.

The highly destructive impact of asbestos is not limited to human health. The tidal wave of lawsuits against asbestos companies is having a significant effect on the American business landscape. More than six hundred thousand lawsuits and claims have been filed by asbestos victims. Juries awarded hundreds of thousands and then millions of dollars in compensatory and punitive damages.

In the wake of this legal avalanche, more than fifty American companies, including Kaiser Aluminum, Owens Corning, and Bethlehem Steel, have filed for protection under Chapter 11 of the Bankruptcy Code, and many more may follow. The bankruptcy filings led to a highly controversial judicial process for handling asbestos claims that is still being used today. They have also led to heavy lobbying in Congress as industry and plaintiff lawyers fight for the billions of dollars that are at stake.

Asbestos is not just an American problem. Asbestos-related diseases will soon be the number one cause of death of European men under the age of sixty-five, according to the Trades Union Congress of the United Kingdom. Official death totals in western Europe may exceed five hundred thousand by the year 2020, according to international asbestos expert Dr. Robin Howie of the British Occupational Hygiene Society. Faced with these overwhelming death tolls, most western European countries have already banned all uses and the export of asbestos.

Globally, the deadly count persists—seventy-five thousand fatalities predicted in Australia, five thousand deaths already in Chile, two victims a day in Scotland, and thousands more in nearly every industrialized country in the world. Asbestos officially kills more than one hundred thousand workers worldwide every year, and that number is expected to increase for decades, according to the United Nations' International Labor Organization.

Asbestos remains legal in much of eastern Europe, where regional studies show death rates among workers outpace even the worse-case scenarios in the West. After the Soviets fell out of power, Polish workers discovered that the masks the Soviet managers had given them to prevent asbestos exposure were actually made of asbestos. Yet official Soviet medical records showed no worker illnesses due to asbestos exposure. Even today, Russia, the world's largest exporter of asbestos, is reluctant to address the issue.

South Africa, which has long been one of the world's largest producers of the most lethal types of asbestos, has a hideous record with the mineral. Dr. Gerrit Schepers, an American doctor visiting South Africa during the apartheid era, told of seeing young Bantu tribal children forced to work at the bottom of huge bags, compressing the asbestos with their feet while blue asbestos was being dumped continuously over their heads. Dr. Schepers doubted if any of the children lived beyond their teenage years.

Huge populations in China—where prison laborers were forced to work the asbestos mines—and in India, Mexico, Southeast Asia, South America, and much of Africa, are being exposed to millions of tons of imported asbestos as the demand in Third World countries has skyrocketed, stoked by the worldwide asbestos industry, which has seen its customer base in the industrialized nations diminish. The lack of occupational and consumer protection laws in these countries will mean increased death rates for generations to come.

While the medical hazards, financial disasters, political failures, and corporate treachery tell a shocking tale in their own right, perhaps the true tragedy of asbestos can be fully understood only through the personal stories of those whose lives have been altered by it.

No community in America is suffering more from asbestos contamination than Libby, Montana. The horrifying events that have taken place there have led to critical breakthroughs in our understanding of asbestos exposure. They have come at a price, though, one that the people in Libby would surely have forgone had they been given the choice.

3

LIBBY'S DEADLY FIELDS

"Libby was a beautiful place to grow up. The town was like a big family. In the summer we used to swim, ride bicycles, and go to baseball games. Nobody ever locked their doors at night. There was very little crime, if you didn't count what W. R. Grace was doing."

—*Gayla Benefield*

When WWII ended, it wasn't Germany or Japan that took over the United States, it was baseball. In the years following the war, household names like Normandy Beach, Anzio, and Midway Island gave way to names like Mickey Mantle, Yogi Berra, and Willie Mays. For young men around the country, ball fields took the place of battlefields. In big cities and small towns, baseball diamonds became the official community centers where families gathered and gossiped and cheered and healed from the wounds of war. Baseball was the dusty, noisy, beating heart of a nation trying to regain its innocence and joy.

As poet William Carlos Williams wrote:

The crowd at the ball game
Is moved uniformly

By a spirit of uselessness
Which delights them.

America believed in the redemption of baseball, and so did the residents of Libby. Fierce rivalries grew up with nearby towns like Troy and Bonners Ferry, and Little League teams came from as far away as Kalispell and Whitefish to play in Libby. Thousands of young ballplayers battled it out on the four diamonds at the north edge of town during the 1960s and 1970s.

There to help during those years, donating bats, balls, gloves, and even waste dirt from the mine for the baseball fields, was W. R. Grace. Grace officials kept a high profile in Libby, lending a helping hand to the community, especially during baseball season. Usually, the local newspapers were there to cover the company's good deeds.

There was only one problem. The baseball diamonds and piles of vermiculite that surrounded Grace's expanding plant by the river were heavily contaminated with an asbestos fiber called tremolite, which has no commercial application but is considered one of the more deadly forms of asbestos.

"I watched games there, my children played there; heck, just everybody who lived here went down to those ball fields at one time or another," said Gayla Benefield. "The children who were too young to play baseball used to play beyond the outfield fence in the piles of vermiculite there. It was worse even than the ball fields. It was filled with asbestos dust."

Benefield and the other Libby residents were completely unaware of the peril. Libby seemed a million miles away from the environmental dangers that plagued the big cities of America.

Benefield was a graduate of Libby High School, where the running track was also highly contaminated with tremolite asbestos from waste dirt donated by Grace. For four decades, every child who ran on the track, which was used for gym classes as well as track meets, was exposed to the deadly tremolite fibers.

In 1965, Gayla married David Benefield, and together they raised five children. Gayla worked for the local power company as a meter reader. David worked as a labor union representative. Life was good, although Gayla worried about her father, Perley. In 1966, he was still working at the mine, but he was suffering frequent chest pains. The company doctor told him bluntly that he could die of a heart attack at any time.

"Grace had X-rayed Dad's chest, like they did just about all the other miners, and when he didn't hear from them, he thought he was fine," said Gayla. "He was shocked and depressed to find out about his heart. The most important thing to him, what he worried about, was whether he could run the company road grader. He always prayed for snow on Christmas because it would mean double time."

The miners who lived in Libby would rise early. Most rode the bus north over the Kootenai River Bridge to Rainy Creek Road, a broad, winding dirt road that took them to the mine. The wives and families were allowed to join the men for lunch at the mine, and many did. On weekends the families often got together for picnics and parties.

"It really was like a big family here," Gayla said. "We all knew each other, of course, and we all felt privileged to be part of the mine."

The sawmill at the east end of Libby often employed more than a thousand people during boom times, but the mine was as close to an elite club as Libby had. The jobs there were coveted. It paid higher salaries than logging, and the work seemed safer than sawing, choking, and hauling heavy timber.

Protected by the big-shouldered Cabinet Mountains to the west, which coaxed the moisture out of most of the storms blown in from Canada, Libby often escaped the savage winter weather that slammed other parts of Montana. Temperatures could plunge to below zero, however, and the men at the mine who worked outside often toiled through thin blankets of snow. Most were used to it. These were tough, self-reliant men, yet they were often awkwardly naive and worldly innocent at the same time. Their wives usually matched them in all those categories. They accepted the fact that many of the workers at the mine died at a relatively early age. Many of the loggers died early, too. It was simply the way life was in Libby.

In 1968, Perley's chest pains worsened and his breathing became increasingly restricted. One day he was called in to the mine office and told he was being taken off the road grader. Perley was frightened that he was going to be fired. He was grateful when they told him he was being transferred to a new position. He knew that he was too sick to get a job anywhere else.

"They gave him a job back in the dry mill, which is where he started," Gayla said with anger. "It was the dustiest place at the mine."

What Perley didn't know was that the mine managers had already listed him as one of the sickest men on their payroll. Their confidential X rays showed he had serious lung burdens and abnormalities.

By 1971, Perley was sick most of the time. Common colds could last months, and he coughed constantly and struggled for breath. The company finally suggested that he file for workers' compensation and retire on disability. What they didn't tell him was that by filing for workers' compensation he would give up his legal rights to sue the company once he learned why he was sick. Perley grew weaker and finally went to a private doctor in Missoula who told him there was nothing wrong with his heart. He was suffering from advanced pulmonary fibrosis.

"We were confused by that," said Gayla. "It was obvious that somebody was lying. Before this we always thought it was the dust that made some of the men at the mines sick. Everybody called it 'white lung disease.' So, why would they say he had heart problems and hide the fact that Dad had a lung disease? That was the first time that red flags went up for me."

Perley's health worsened quickly after that. He coughed incessantly. The worst part was that Perley finally knew he had been betrayed by the company to which he had given his loyalty and so many years of his life.

"He just couldn't understand it," Gayla said. "It hurt him deep down."

By the time he was sixty-one years old, Perley couldn't walk outside to the garage. "This is a man who was willing to work eighteen hours in the snow at Christmas because it meant more money for his family," Gayla said. "He died quietly. He just didn't have the will to fight anymore."

Bob Wilkins never got used to the men dying early at the mine. "When it happened, the company usually blamed it on the fact that so many of the men smoked, but I never got used to losing so many friends," he said.

Still, for those who remained, life was good in Libby. Wilkins loved the wildness of the forests and mountains surrounding the little valley. Nearly every weekend he took his family hiking and camping into the nearby Cabinet Wilderness Area. The thick-timbered Rocky Mountains were home to moose, elk, white-tailed deer, bear, fox, and a menagerie of other wildlife. On the rocky cliffs, families of bighorn sheep would appear in the late afternoons, the lambs sending rocks clattering down the sheer precipices. In the summers, the canyons were lit long into the evening by an arctic half-light that ran with the rhythm of Libby Creek on its way to meet the Kootenai.

For Wilkins, the time brought a tranquillity he had never known. Growing up in Memphis, Tennessee, he did well in school and graduated from high school when he was sixteen years old. His friends, who were all eighteen, were caught up in the patriotic fever of 1941 and joined the army. Wilkins talked his mother into faking his age on the recruitment papers and joined with them. When the war broke out, he was transferred to the air force and served in the South Seas, seeing frequent combat.

Later, after the war, his job as police chief in Wolf Point had also brought him, on occasion, face-to-face with the violence that men can do. It was in the soft light of the canyons near Libby that Wilkins finally believed he had found peace. He loved spending time with his family. They fished and packed in picnic lunches, and in the summers swam in the pure waters of the Kootenai. Wilkins was proud of his job, and he was quick to agree when the company asked him to help fix the baseball fields and the nearby running track.

"We brought down waste material, which was mostly a mix of dirt and vermiculite, and put it down on top of everything," he recalled. "We spread it out and even built the baseball bleachers right on top of it. None of the workers knew that it was contaminated with asbestos. But the company knew—and nobody said a word."

The company also donated dirt from the mine for the town skating rink and the running track at the Libby middle school. Defense attorneys would later argue that these donations proved Grace officials did not know that the material was polluted with the killer fibers. How could any company, they asked, be so cold-blooded as to do that?

What Wilkins and the other employees of the mine did not know was that the Montana Board of Health had been long concerned about the health hazards of the dust. According to Montana Department of Environmental Quality records, the state conducted an inspection of the mine on December 9, 1941, and found that dust levels were high throughout the mine. At the time, it was producing about twenty thousand tons of vermiculite per year. The State Board of Health requested that workers loading materials be required to wear respirators. The Universal Zonolite Insulation Company, which owned the mine at that time, responded by installing exhaust ventilation fans to help with the dust.

In 1955, after the company had streamlined its name to the Zonolite Company, Ben Wake, an industrial hygiene engineer for the Division of Disease Prevention and Control for the State of Montana, became concerned about the high potential for pneumoconiosis in the Libby miners, a condition in which deposits collect in the lungs. Wake was also concerned about the composition of the vermiculite, but his requests to have it analyzed by federal researchers were repeatedly ignored.

In 1956, asbestos was officially listed as an ingredient of the dust at the mine. Wake's report on the mine indicated that company records showed the asbestos content of the dust to be from 8 percent to 21 percent. He recommended further improvements to the ventilation system and stated that use of respirators in the dry milling process be mandatory.

Wake again sent samples of the vermiculite to be analyzed. This time he received a letter from Dohrman Byers, an official with the then-federal Department of Health, Education and Welfare. Byers told Wake that the government did not yet have a reliable method to determine asbestos in the samples. "However," Byers wrote, "if the company will cooperate and control the dust, the asbestosis and silicosis hazard would certainly be minimal."

The language in Byers's letter was critical. It seems to indicate that the government and the mine owners were well aware of the fact that asbestos caused asbestosis and that asbestos was present and a hazard at the mine long before W. R. Grace purchased it. Despite this knowledge, the miners were not told of the asbestos dangers.

Les Skramstad remembered that the mine managers did hand out flimsy paper masks to the miners. "None of us ever wore the things," Skramstad said. "It turns out they were useless against stopping asbestos fibers anyway. There were other, better, respirators, but they clogged up with dust after a few minutes and we never wore those either. The word 'asbestos' was never mentioned by anybody at the mine. All we were told is that it was a nuisance dust and that you breathed it in and you would exhale it right back out."

The dust was omnipresent at the mine. "I remember it blocked out the light to the point I would sometimes walk right into the support beams," Skramstad said. "My nose would get packed with that dust. It was mighty hard to breathe."

Wake inspected the mine again in 1959. According to his report, he found that in some areas of the mine the dust was 27 percent asbestos. His report was not shared with the miners. Court cases would later show that in 1959, more than one-third of workers at the vermiculite mine in Libby had chest X rays that were abnormal. In 1962, another important discovery was exposed in Wake's growing pile of reports when he mentioned that tremolite was a known contaminate of the vermiculite. Wake sent air and ore samples from the mine and a series of questions to the federal Occupations Health Research Facility in Ohio for analysis and received these results:

- To determine if asbestos is present in the ore—Yes.
- Type of asbestos—tremolite.
- Percent of asbestos fibers in airborne dust samples—
  40 percent.

Wake concluded that the company had made no progress in reducing dust concentration in the dry mill. He also insisted that the classification of the dust be changed. "It is no longer nuisance dust because of vermiculite mining, but should be classified in the same category as talc, and asbestos content should be closely observed." Wake's official change never made its way to the mine. It was called a "nuisance dust" by mine managers until the mine closed in 1990.

In 1963, the year Grace bought the mine, Wake reported that an analysis of the vermiculite at the mine "indicated 6.2 percent to 22.5 percent tremolite present." The following year, at the request of the Local Union 361 leadership, Wake returned to the mine and recommended a number of housekeeping improvements to cut down on the dust. The mine was found out of compliance with dust regulations in a number of areas, but no enforcement procedures were taken against Grace by any governmental agency. The union leadership remained unhappy but never had enough leverage to do anything about it.

"There were so many other guys around town who would have taken our jobs in an instant, we couldn't push Grace very hard," said Wilkins, who was the president of Local 361 in the late 1970s. "Hell, the federal and state governments weren't doing anything to stop Grace, how could we?"

How much the company knew and when they knew it is clearly delineated in a confidential November 25, 1967, letter from S. Y. Larrick, a Grace executive, to John Hopkins, an official with the mine's insurer, Maryland Casualty Company. Larrick, who referred to W. R. Grace as the "insured" throughout the letter, initially addressed the State Board of Health's 1956 concerns about the dust.

"The plant inspections did reveal asbestos content, and of

course the percentage of such fibers found to exist in the dust in the mill did far exceed what were considered to be allowable concentrations," he wrote. "Many recommendations were presented by the State Board and it would appear that the insured gradually attempted to correct the situation. It must, however, further be considered that it might appear to others that the action taken by the insured to correct the situation, might not, to the unbiased observer, appear to have been either extremely effective, or quickly performed."

Larrick's letter continued, "In 1962, dust samples revealed a high asbestos content and the State Board's conclusions, at the time, were that 'No progress had been made in reducing the dust concentrations in the dry mill to an acceptable level, and that indeed the dust concentrations had been increased substantially.' . . . In 1963, concentrations again were determined to be well in excess of acceptable levels."

Larrick then suggested that Grace follow the strategy that Johns-Manville had pioneered nearly thirty years before. "As I informed you, I would hesitate to allow in evidence the State Board reports if it is possible to keep them out of the hands of the Industrial Accident Board, and through it, the general public. While I have not researched the problem, it has even occurred to me that the insured's inability to curb the problems regarding the State's Board's recommendations through the years, might be alleged at least to have constituted willful and wanton conduct on its part, with whatever complications that particular charge might carry with it."

The letter then plunges ever deeper into an industry defense attorney's nightmare.

Further, Mr. [Earl] Lovick [Grace mine manager], for the first time, thought to advise me of certain studies which have been conducted by a local radiologist since around 1963 or 1964, which apparently have involved obtaining

annual X-rays of all employees for study. The information
furnished by Mr. Lovick was to the effect that the radiolo-
gist was convinced that a good many of the employees suf-
fered from lung abnormalities which could be the result of
encroaching asbestosis. This information of course appeared
to me to be of extreme importance, and we made arrange-
ments to travel to Whitefish, Montana, immediately to
interview the radiologist. The radiologist involved, Dr.
William Little, informed me that his studies most certainly
did indicate there to be present a great deal of lung abnor-
malities among the employees, far in excess of the percentage
one would find in examining the ordinary population, and
he did in addition point out that the situation was even
more severe, when considering he was in general examining
young, hearty male workmen. Dr. Little stated that we did
indeed have a severe problem, and that we might expect a
good many claims involving asbestosis.

The most incendiary part of the letter was contained in Larrick's next paragraph:

We might point out that apparently the only persons aware
of the studies are the insured's officials and Dr. Little. Again,
as you may well realize, I would much like to avoid having
evidence presented by the opposing party which would re-
veal the extent and severity of the problem with which we
are concerned.

The enormity of the cover-up would be hard to believe if it
hadn't happened in so many asbestos-related cases around the
world. Larrick's letter exposed the fact that not only did the mine
manager know about the health problems, but the insurance company, the radiologist, and the State of Montana certainly knew of the

potential for this type of widespread disease. None of these parties informed the miners.

In a foreshadowing of the tragedy to come in Libby, Larrick noted that studies had shown that the asbestos contamination was not limited to the dry mill. "The fact also now must be considered that a great many of the employees suffer from lung abnormalities and a good many of them have probably never been in the mill, which of course simply means that they are contracting the disease in the yard or in fact at any point where a dust condition may exist," he wrote.

There was no mention in his letter about the dust condition that existed at the popping plant at the north edge of town between the baseball fields, but it is hard to believe that the company was unable to extend Larrick's warning to that area as well.

By 1971, the mine was roaring in full production, yielding more than two hundred thousand tons of vermiculite annually, about 80 percent of the world's total. The company had installed new ventilation systems that helped eliminate the indoor dust. Drills with bag houses were also used to decrease the dust problems. Later, the company would claim it spent more than $14 million on occupational safety problems.

The operation, however, had to move and crush about fifteen thousand tons of ore per day to produce one ton of concentrated vermiculite, and the ever-busy smokestacks were blowing out five thousand tons of dust and fibers per day. The state conducted another inspection that year and determined:

• The bottom-floor operator and two sweepers were exposed to seven times the threshold limit value for asbestos.

- The dust level on the sixth floor of the dry mill was "too dense to count."
- The electrician's exposure was six times the safety limit.
- The loading dock foreman suffered a "very high" exposure, as did all those who rode the contaminated bus to and from work.
- More than twenty other workers were found to have elevated levels of exposure.

Despite these violations, no disciplinary or enforcement action was taken against the mine by the state. Reports showed the company was let off the hook because it had scheduled a new "wet mill" for construction that the company promised would reduce fiber counts.

As the problems with the asbestos exposure mounted for Grace, the company executives began to turn increasingly to Johns-Manville for help. As early as 1967, Grace officials at Libby and J-M environmental control experts corresponded over the dust problem in Libby. On December 26, Grace representative Peter Kostie met with two directors of J-M's environmental control department in Manville. Ten days later, on January 5, 1968, Kostie, in a confidential, intracompany memo to a Zonolite official, R. W. Sterrett in Chicago, outlined "some of the things that came out of the meeting." (At the time, there were thirty-two men at the Libby mine whose X rays showed significant abnormalities.)

"After it is recognized that we do have dust problems and the problem areas are identified," Kostie wrote, "we should move as fast in doing whatever has to be done to remedy the situation. This is of course to minimize dust inhalation by all employees, but most im-

portant to arrest lung contamination by the thirty-two aforemen-
tioned employees. These employees, as far as we know, are not
presently disabled. If we minimize their exposure . . . chances are we
may be able to keep them on the job until they retire, thus pre-
cluding the high cost of total disability." The letter is chilling in its
implications, and a clear indication of how J-M executives, and now
Grace officials, had come to view the "asbestos problem."

Nowhere in Kostie's letter was there any expression of concern
from either him or the J-M officials about the miners being exposed
to additional fibers. The tenor of the letter is exemplified in this passage from Kostie:

"They [J-M industrial hygiene experts] apparently feel that any
exposure to asbestos dust is hazardous. Many doctors are of the
opinion that there is a definite relationship between asbestos dust
and certain types of cancer. J-M anticipates that every cancer case
among their employees will be a potential Workmen's Compensation case."

The J-M officials also recommended that Grace settle a claim
from a former employee who suffered from advanced lung disease.
"Public relations could be damaged otherwise," Kostie wrote.

At the end of the letter, Kostie recommended that J-M be contracted to do further work for Grace regarding the asbestos fallout.
Grace would follow many of J-M's strategies for the next thirty-five
years.

One of these strategies was something that can be called the "promotable villain." It is still often used by public relations companies
and political and corporate spin-makers when they need to do
damage control. The goal is to deflect attention from an issue for
which a client or company is being criticized. The key is to find a de-

spicable villain associated with the issue, however remotely, that makes all other problems—especially the one associated with you— seem mild by comparison. For example, it is almost a tradition for American presidents, when facing drooping poll numbers due to a domestic or economic crisis, to find a foreign tyrant who needs a good thrashing. It is a fairly simple task to find a promotable villain among today's petty despots, and an air strike or two invariably brings the president's approval ratings back up.

The asbestos companies, led by J-M, had already focused on one of the most promotable villains in the country—the tobacco industry. When miners and workers who smoked came down with lung cancer, the disease was always written off to the tobacco use. Many of the asbestos companies underwent fierce campaigns to reduce tobacco use in their plants, even as they did nothing to curb asbestos exposure.

In 1977, J-M consultants helped Earl Lovick and the other mine officials develop a program of employee education concerning the asbestos health hazards. In a classic maneuver, the company determined that at the time the program was announced, it would also announce a ban on smoking at the mine. They assumed correctly that the smoking ban would grab the attention of most of the miners and the media, deflecting concerns away from the asbestos problem.

One of the key elements of the program was a slide show to be given to the miners. J-M provided much of the script of the slide show. It was little more than a public relations scam, riddled with inaccuracies. For example, the suggested commentary on a slide about mesothelioma included this: "Recent studies indicate that asbestos is not the only cause that might increase the risk of this disease. There are many cases of mesothelioma among people who have no history of exposure to asbestos fiber." The commentary does not include any examples because the majority of medical experts believe mesothelioma is caused only by asbestos fibers.

The slide show also indicated that the body's defense system filters out asbestos fibers by eating them. It was this section that later inspired Wilkins, who watched the premiere of the slide show at the mine, to create a T-shirt that read: ASBESTOS: PUT A LITTLE FIBER IN YOUR DIET.

"Substances that manage to escape the body's defense system then are subject to attack by special cells," the commentary promised. "They surround and render virtually harmless most invading particles." At that time, roughly a quarter of the men watching the slide show had abnormal lung X rays. Many more would develop asbestosis and lung cancer in the coming years.

The next slide showed a villainous cigarette being snuffed out. "Again," the commentator said, "we must emphasize the dangers of smoking."

The commentator promised the men that they would be notified in the unlikely event that fiber exposure levels were ever exceeded, and respirators would be made available. Wilkins laughed until he began coughing when he recalled the words. "Those were just bald-faced lies," he said. "We weren't ever told anything except not to smoke."

The company saved the best for last. "Don't take chances with your health," the script concluded. "We don't want you to."

The employees were told shortly thereafter that out of a total of 197 chest X rays taken at the mine, 25 percent showed abnormalities. The company blamed the problems on smoking. In a confidential company memo, Lovick wrote: "It was stated that in almost all of these cases where abnormal chests were shown, with a few exceptions, the people who showed abnormalities in their X-rays were smokers." Lovick added that the company had also issued a policy that it would "no longer hire a person who smokes tobacco."

During that time the asbestos industry had full knowledge that the deadly fallout from their product wasn't just contained to their mines and manufacturing plants. Legal documents would later show that, by the mid-1970s, coldly calculated actuarial tables were being developed to consider the deaths of not only the employees but their families as well.

In March 1977, a report developed for the insurance industry called the asbestos problem a "catastrophe" for asbestos and insurance companies. It calculated that there would be at least four hundred thousand potential plaintiffs. "This figure does not take into account consideration of 'other' possible cancer victims of asbestosis such as wives of workers, persons living near asbestos factories, school children, etc.," the report stated. Insurance company documents also recognized that there "exists the potential claim from the wives or homemakers of those asbestos workers. The wife becomes exposed to the dust where she handles and cleans the clothes containing the dust particles."

That information, for whatever reason, never reached the people of Libby.

About the time that Grace began its "employee education program" at the mine, the company was allowing vermiculite to be spread throughout the town. It was being used in homes, in school yards, and on roadways. Like Gayla Benefield's mother, Margaret, wives and family members of the miners were beginning to suffer from respiratory problems that they couldn't seem to shake. By 1978,

Margaret was coughing all the time and her chest ached. The poison that had killed Perley was now bearing down on her.

"We thought Mom and some of the others just had a bad case of pneumonia," said Gayla. "We just didn't know anything, yet. We were naive and trusting. At that time I was still raising my kids, and we were still going to the ballpark every spring and summer. We didn't know that every time a player slid into a base it raised fibers into the air, or that the younger kids were being exposed every time they played on the vermiculite piles they had by the popping plant. Baseball was our major sport in Libby. For a lot of families, it was their happiest time, going down to the ballpark to watch the games and chat with their neighbors. That's what Libby was all about."

At the time, that is what much of America was all about. The difference was that in Libby there was no such thing as being safe at home.

4

THE DISEASE OF SLAVES

Billy Poch had never been so proud. The eighth grader was touring the impressive collection of sixteen huge buildings that made up the Johns-Manville Company Plant in the town named after the company, Manville, New Jersey. He couldn't wait until his class reached Building 8. That's where his dad, Bill Sr., worked, cleaning what was called the Dust House.

The year was 1939, and violent events in Europe had everyone talking about the possibility of war. Johns-Manville, the largest producer of asbestos products in America, was developing a number of products for the United States military. When he and his friends walked through the Dust House, Poch felt a rush of pride that his parents worked for such a company. He was also amazed at the amount of dust that seemed to be everywhere in the plant. His mother, Alice, who worked at the plant too, met him at lunchtime.

"How did you like Johns-Manville?" she asked in her heavily accented English. Like the Pochs, most of the workers at the Manville plant were immigrants from Hungary and other eastern and middle European countries. Most of them spoke little English and felt lucky to find work.

Poch shook his head. "Mom, I hope I never work here," he

said. "I would hate to work in all that dust. Everyone in the plant seemed like they were covered in it."

To Bill and Alice Poch, the jobs at the J-M plant had been a godsend. Together they made just seven dollars a week, but it meant they could provide for their family.

Poch looked forward to late afternoon when his parents would come home. His father would grab his young son in his arms and carry him through the house, asking him about his day. All the workers wore wool clothing, and Bill Sr.'s shirt and pants would be covered with white dust.

If the Pochs felt lucky to have jobs at the plant, Joe Utasi was ecstatic. His father had emigrated from Hungary in the 1920s and found work in the West Virginia coal mines, where he suffered a back injury in the early 1930s. With his father unable to work, the family ended up in New Jersey, destitute and on welfare.

"There were six kids in the family and we all grew up eating soup and potatoes," Utasi recalled. "My mom would get bread from somewhere, but she'd have to scrape the mold off it and heat it up before we could eat it. There weren't any fruit or vegetables in our house; milk was a holiday thing. But it was almost as bad with every other family in town."

When he was sixteen, Utasi went to the J-M plant to look for work. It was six o'clock in the morning when he got there. He was shocked to see about four hundred people squatting in the grass, waiting for the boss to come out and pick the dozen or so lucky ones who would be chosen to work that day. Utasi was thrilled when the boss pointed at him. He vowed to survive the miserable jobs they gave him. The gregarious teenager worked hard, and soon he was given a full-time position at forty-five cents an hour.

Everybody liked the teenage Utasi because even though he

did one of the foulest jobs in the plant, including shoveling broken asbestos shingles into a dusty grinder, he always wore a smile. He would laugh whenever they teased him about the wooden shoes he had to wear because the metal floor surrounding the asbestos grinder got so hot.

"It was dusty all the time in the plant, sometimes the lightbulbs were just white blurs in the room," he recalled. "But in the 1930s, complaining about working conditions was something that few of us dared do. Not with four hundred hungry people sitting outside on the lawn ready and willing to do our jobs."

Most of us logically assume that any substance as dangerous as asbestos would have long ago been ferreted out by government regulators and activists. Yet, for a number of reasons, that has not happened. Many of these reasons are embedded deep within the tortured history of asbestos, which Paul Brodeur, an investigative reporter for *The New Yorker*, once characterized as "a history of corporate malfeasance and inhumanity to man that is unparalleled in the annals of the private-enterprise system." To understand the current threat and costs of asbestos, it is critical to understand its history, which began when miners first extracted the mineral from the earth and let the genie out of the bottle.

The Roman historian Pliny the Elder wrote about the astonishing "magic mineral" that resisted fire and was so delicate it could be woven and spun as easily as cotton or flax fibers. The Romans were especially impressed by the fact that even when exposed to the fiercest fire, asbestos garments came out whiter than before. The Latin word for asbestos, *amiantus*, translates roughly to "unpolluted." But the Romans also knew of its dangers and delegated the asbestos work accordingly. They called asbestosis the "disease of slaves."

Finnish potters used asbestos twenty-five hundred years ago as a binding and strengthening agent as well as for its fire-resistant qualities. The ancient Greeks were also fascinated by the material that wouldn't burn. Asbestos, in Greek, means "inextinguishable."

Interest in asbestos died down after that, although Marco Polo was said to have been introduced to it during his travels in Asia. Its modern uses were rediscovered in the 1870s, when the first asbestos mines in the world were opened near the small Canadian town of Thetford, in the Quebec Province. A large deposit of white asbestos, called chrysotile (*kris-o-til*), was mined by the hundreds of tons. More than 95 percent of all asbestos products are made of chrysotile, which is most often formed in serpentine, a finely grained rock made of water-bearing magnesium silicates. The asbestos is separated from the ore body through crushing, air suction, and vibrating screens. The process inevitably creates a massive amount of asbestos-laden dust.

Once the multitude of commercial uses for asbestos was realized, demand grew quickly. In 1897, there were reports of "hundreds of buildings plastered with asbestic" in New York City, and by the early 1900s, the annual world production of asbestos had grown to more than thirty thousand tons. Along with the boom in mining and manufacturing of asbestos came a trickle of troubling reports of pulmonary diseases among asbestos workers. By 1897, an Italian medical study had already labeled asbestos dust as the cause of an outbreak of lung disease among asbestos weavers and their families.

It is probable that a young man named Henry Ward Johns was not aware of these reports when he founded and built a company in lower Manhattan in the late 1850s to sell the new roofing material he had patented. Made of burlap, asbestos, tar, and a few other ingredients, Johns boasted that he could make a home fireproof. Demand for his unique product grew, and before long the H. W. Johns Manufacturing Company was a thriving enterprise.

Later, when the company merged with the Manville Corporation to become the Johns-Manville Company, it would become the largest asbestos manufacturer in the United States. Johns died in 1898, a probable victim of his own product. His official cause of death was "dust phthisis pneumonitis," which was almost certainly asbestosis.

From 1899 through 1910, British factory inspectors filed a number of reports relating the manufacture of asbestos to "injury to the bronchial tubes and lungs." In 1900—one hundred years before the events at Libby burst into the headlines—Dr. Montague Murray, who worked at the Charing Cross Hospital in London, performed an autopsy on a British asbestos worker. Before he died of pulmonary failure, the worker told inspectors that he was the last survivor out of ten people working in the company's carding room, where the asbestos was separated and purified by hand. The autopsy showed that the victim, who died at age thirty-three, had a massive number of asbestos fibers in his lungs. It marked the first time asbestos was officially tied to the death of a worker.

In 1906, an English factory inspector near London wrote: "Of all the injurious dusty processes of which I have again received complaints, none, I believe, surpass in injuriousness to the workers the sieving, preparing, carding, and spinning processes in asbestos manufacture."

There were also continuing public reports of worker deaths from "fibrosis" in asbestos plants in Italy and France during this time. Ten years later, studies in the United States began showing that asbestos workers were dying unnaturally young. The studies were conclusive to the point that some American and Canadian insurance companies began refusing to issue life insurance policies to asbestos workers.

The first official case where the term *asbestosis* was used in medical literature was reported in 1924 in England. A British physician, Dr. W. E. Cooke, conducted an autopsy on a thirty-three-year-old woman who had died of lung problems after working in an asbestos-textile factory from the age of thirteen. The classic signs of asbestosis were evident, including extensive pulmonary fibrosis and damaged lungs and pleural membranes. The study was reported in the *British Medical Journal*, which set off a flurry of interest in asbestos within the medical community in England.

A number of studies followed, including a critical 1929 study by a chief English medical inspector, Dr. E. R. A. Merewether, of 363 asbestos-textile workers in Britain, according to Brodeur in his book *Outrageous Misconduct: The Asbestos Industry on Trial* (Pantheon, 1985). Dr. Merewether found that more than 25 percent of the workers showed evidence of pulmonary fibrosis. He also found that there was a significant relationship between the percentage of incidence among the workers and the number of years they had been employed. More than 80 percent of those who had been employed for more than twenty years were afflicted.

During this time, no significant studies on asbestos were done by the American Medical Association or by any U.S. governmental health agency. The first workman's compensation claim regarding asbestos, however, was filed in an asbestos-textile mill in Massachusetts in 1927. It was upheld in subsequent challenges, and in 1930, the first official case of asbestosis in the United States was reported in the journal *Minnesota Medicine*. The report was then published in the *Journal of the American Medical Association*, which was mailed directly to nearly half the doctors in the United States. That same year, a man exposed to asbestos while doing maintenance work in a government hospital was officially diagnosed and received compensation for his disability.

In 1931, England enacted laws to regulate asbestos levels in factories, and in 1932, *Encyclopedia Britannica* identified asbestos fibers as a cause of lung cancer. By then, most companies, especially those in the asbestos industry, were well aware that the dust in the mines and factories was unhealthy for their workers. That understanding made the events that followed in Manville, New Jersey, even more astonishing.

It is probable that few if any of the thousands of workers in the Manville plant in the 1930s had ever heard of a man named Sumner Simpson. He didn't work for Johns-Manville, but he would play a significant role in their future as well as the future of asbestos workers for generations to come.

Simpson was, like William Russell Grace before him, a larger-than-life industrial entrepreneur. He came out of Bridgeport, Connecticut, bent on making a fortune in the wide-open markets of the 1920s. Noting the burgeoning interest and sales of automobiles, Simpson founded the Raybestos Company and began manufacturing and selling asbestos brake linings and clutch parts. In 1929, Simpson went to New York and merged his company with the Manhattan Rubber Manufacturing Company and with the United States Asbestos Company in Manheim, Pennsylvania. He renamed his new conglomerate the Raybestos-Manhattan Company.

At the same time, an ambitious Iowan named Lewis H. Brown was about to take over the helm of Johns-Manville. The course he would set, with Simpson's help, would prove highly profitable during their lifetimes. It would also ultimately plunge both companies down the path to ruin, wreak havoc among dozens of other national and multinational companies, and lead to the untimely deaths of tens of thousands of unsuspecting workers.

Lewis Brown was a strikingly handsome man; he could have been a leading man, with his pencil-thin mustache, fine features, and firm jaw. His actions, however, would ultimately speak more clearly than anything else about the quality of his character.

Brown, and his brother, Vandiver Brown, who served as chief counsel to Johns-Manville, did generate goodwill among his employees by adopting a forty-hour workweek and by insisting on periodic physical examinations for all workers, including, in the case of asbestos workers, periodic chest X rays—a practice that would come back to haunt the company forty years later.

By the early 1930s, not long after the Browns gained control of Johns-Manville, they had access to a number of reports indicating that asbestos dust was a significant danger to workers at both Johns-Manville and Raybestos-Manhattan. It was also clear that they were deeply concerned about how future workers' compensation issues might affect their companies. In 1933, lawsuits brought by workers in different companies who suffered lung disease from "silicosis," which was called the "Depression Disease," and undoubtedly included some asbestosis victims, totaled $100 million. The number would jump to $300 million the following year.

By 1932, many insurance companies had already opted out of insuring most asbestos workers. Brodeur, in *Outrageous Misconduct*, noted that a 1932 letter from the United States Bureau of Mines to asbestos manufacturer Eagle-Picher stated: "It is now known that asbestos dust is one of the most dangerous dusts to which man is exposed."

A number of industry association publications followed with stories on the adverse health effects of asbestos and called for worker protections in the form of dust masks and dust control. These included an occupational disease report in 1932, published in *National Underwriter* magazine, that concluded: "Any processes involving asbestos are considered especially hazardous, for the asbestos fibers appear to be difficult to expel from the lungs." Two years prior, the

Journal of the American Medical Association wrote, "Asbestos is mined and manufactured in many parts of the country and . . . pulmonary asbestosis surely will be encountered."

What few people knew at the time, however, was that from October 1929 to January 1931, the asbestos industry asked the Metropolitan Life Insurance Company to do a medical study on asbestos worker fatalities in several textile plants. The team, led by Dr. Anthony Lanza, a medical doctor who worked for the Metropolitan Life Insurance Company, also took chest X rays of 126 workers who had been employed for more than three years. The report confirmed Brown's and Simpson's worst fears. Dr. Lanza found that 67 of the workers had already developed asbestosis and 39 of them had scarring and other preliminary signs of the disease. Dr. Lanza and his team recommended that Johns-Manville and Raybestos-Manhattan find ways to greatly reduce the asbestos exposure in the plants. According to the company's attorneys years later, Johns-Manville did carry out all of Dr. Lanza's recommendations. They blamed the continuing health problems on the fact that the federal government's workplace asbestos fiber limits were too high. Plaintiff lawyers disagreed, saying that Dr. Lanza's report, when it was finally published, was greatly watered down and the workers were not properly informed.

At the time Dr. Lanza's report was completed, Johns-Manville was being sued for negligence by eleven workers who were already suffering from asbestosis. The complaints were quickly settled by the company—one of the provisions of the deal was that the plaintiff lawyers could not bring another asbestos suit against the company for ten years—but there was no doubt that Brown and Simpson now greatly feared that future asbestos claims could cause significant financial damage to their companies. According to Brodeur, Dr. Lanza later said that the potential for more legal action "confused and terrified the industrialists and insurance officials" and inspired "dread among them."

Industrial dust, silicosis, asbestos exposure, and "lung fibrosis" problems in the workplace became topics discussed with increasing frequency at national insurance conferences and in insurance-industry journals. In 1935, the *Eastern Underwriter* reported on a keynote speech given at the Annual Convention of the International Association of Industrial Accident Boards and Commissions. The publication quoted T. M. Bartlett, a member of the Advisory Committee of the National Association of Casualty and Surety Executives, as calling the flurry of lawsuits against asbestos companies an "unwholesome situation" that, he said, was "precipitated by disease caused by breathing inorganic dust, particularly the diseases of silicosis and asbestosis. . . . These are not new diseases, but they have been alarmingly on the increase because of exposure to and the use of modern machinery and processes."

In 1935, Brown wrote to Simpson: "I quite agree with you that our interests are best served by having asbestosis receive the minimum of publicity." They took the first step by instructing the editor of *Asbestos Magazine* to publish nothing about asbestosis or the other dangers of asbestos fibers. By then, the written memos between Lewis Brown and Sumner Simpson had become the "smoking gun" that plaintiff attorneys would reference in their legal wars against the asbestos industries. (Simpson, much to the chagrin of the future defense lawyers, was a pack rat and saved the letters as well as other incriminating documents.)

In spite of their censorship efforts, Simpson and Brown felt they had a crisis on their hands in the winter of 1936. Additional asbestos claims were being filed against the companies, and Simpson began writing voluminous letters to his carrier, Metropolitan Life, begging and cajoling the company for more legal protection. In a search for some defendable medical "high" ground, Simpson agreed to allow the U.S. Public Health Service to take chest X rays of employees at the company's South Carolina plant, but only after he gained the hedge he needed. The X rays could be taken only if the government health officials agreed not to share the results with anyone but their own researchers, he insisted. Thus began the strategy that some asbestos companies would emulate for decades. Annual X rays of the asbestos workers were taken—this was usually done by the companies' own doctors—but the results were often withheld from the workers.

At the same time, Vandiver Brown, on behalf of the major companies that largely made up the asbestos industry and which were seeking some sort of medical evidence supporting the industry that they could use in court, contacted Saranac Laboratories in upstate New York, which at the time was one of the nation's leading research centers on industrial pulmonary diseases. Brown first carefully dangled the enticement—Saranac Laboratories would receive funding from the asbestos industry to do animal experiments on asbestos—then he played his trump card. The funding would be available only if those conducting the experiments agreed not to publish the results without the consent of those paying for the experiments. The deal was made, much to the later regret of the chief laboratory scientist. According to Brodeur, he would reveal to a colleague nearly ten years later that most of the test animals exposed to asbestos dust suffered pulmonary diseases. Yet Saranac Labs stuck to its agreement, and the results of the tests were not made public.

Concern over asbestos-related diseases peaked around 1940. Scores of articles in a variety of magazines and newspapers—most of

them trade publications—had already been published, and asbestos legal suits and workers' compensation claims were not un-
common.

By this time, asbestos had become a major product ingredient
around the world. World production had grown from thirty thousand tons in 1901 to five hundred thousand tons in the mid-1930s.

Even as asbestos exposure among workers increased in the
early 1940s, two forces conspired to keep the problem away from
public consciousness. First, the Japanese attack on Pearl Harbor
completely diverted America's attention to the war. Complaining
about work conditions at home—especially within companies
like Johns-Manville, which were contributing greatly to the war
effort—was considered not only unpatriotic but nearly trea-
sonous.

Any hope that the U.S. government would step in to help
curb asbestos exposures in the workplace was tossed aside when
the government itself began using asbestos in great quantities. In
1934, when a passenger ship, the *Morro Castle*, caught fire, re-
sulting in a severe loss of life, the maritime industry began clam-
oring for increased use of asbestos throughout passenger ships and
other vessels. A series of hearings before the U.S. Senate, where few
of the medical studies showing the adverse health effects of asbestos were aired, led to the widespread use of asbestos on all
ships.

With the outbreak of WWII, the U.S. Navy called for large
quantities of asbestos to be used aboard American warships. The
navy's fleet grew from about four hundred ships in 1939 to nearly
sixty-eight hundred ships in 1945. Most contained asbestos to insu-
late pipes, boilers, engines, turbines, and other frictional parts. Asbestos sprays were also used in many ships to help fireproof the
hulls. Working conditions in the shipyards, where an estimated 4.5
million workers were exposed to asbestos, were often worse than

they were in the civilian asbestos plants at Johns-Manville and else-where. The government was in no mood, and no position, to im-pose sanctions on American asbestos corporations.

At the same time, the asbestos industry, led by Johns-Manville and Raybestos-Manhattan, continued its strategy of information control. As a result, the public's concerns over asbestos exposure all but disappeared in the 1940s. It became, once again, the "miracle mineral," and the asbestos industry moved forward, more profitable than ever.

If there is one story that reveals the corporate attitude toward as-bestos workers that still prevails in many areas around the world today, it is the one that took place at the Johns-Manville corpo-rate headquarters in New York City in the months following the attack on Pearl Harbor. The information about the extraordinary meeting that took place there comes from the deposition of Charles H. Roemer, taken April 25, 1984, and reported by Barry Castleman.

In the early 1940s, Charles H. Roemer was an attorney in Pa-terson, New Jersey. His cousin, Dr. Jacob Roemer, had done a study of the workers at the Union Asbestos and Rubber Company's Pa-terson plant and found that a high percentage of them suffered from signs of asbestos disease. Charles Roemer went immediately to the plant manager (who would later die of mesothelioma) and together they set up a meeting with Vandiver and Lewis Brown at the New York headquarters.

Roemer asked the Browns if the physical examination records of their asbestos workers reflected similar findings. Vandiver Brown admitted that X-ray evidence did show that the J-M workers were suffering from a host of asbestos-related lung problems. According to Roemer, Vandiver then told him he would be a fool, though, if he shared the information with the workers. "If our workers are told, they'll stop working and file claims against Johns-Manville," Vandiver said. Looking Roemer straight in the eye, he said that it was the company's policy to let workers continue on the job until they quit work because of asbestosis or died of other asbestos-related disease.

Roemer couldn't believe it. "Do you mean to tell me you would let them work until they dropped dead?" he asked.

"Yes," Brown replied. "We save a lot of money that way."

Roemer was then asked, during his deposition, whether he remembered at what time of the day the meeting took place. He said it was just before noon because he had lunch with the Browns in their boardroom after the meeting.

"I see," said the attorney. "Why do you recall the lunch so vividly?"

"It was the first time in my life I had lobster for lunch," answered Roemer.

Joe Utasi ate his lunch from a lunch pail while sitting on a metal chair, next to the machine that ground up asbestos shingles. "Heck, we didn't know any different," he said. "We never had any protective gear or anything. The dust got everywhere. It was on our eyelids, stuck to the hair on our arms, in the cuffs of your pants, inside your shirt. We never knew it was dangerous."

Utasi met his future wife, Stella, at the J-M plant in the early 1940s. Her job was twisting asbestos with her hands around a copper wire. "We called it yarn," she said. "I remember after we got married, Joe and I would come home with dust all over us. We had to brush it off before we could even come in the house."

As the town of Manville grew up around the prospering J-M

plant, the company worked hard at keeping up good public relations with the community.

"Oh, they helped with everything," recalled Joe. "They donated baseball fields to the town, and they even furnished the bats and balls. We had picnics out there during the summertime. We thought they were wonderful."

Often, the plant blew tons of dust out of its smokestacks, which covered the town. "All the lawns were white; it looked like it had been snowing," said Joe. "We didn't care. We thought the company was so generous because employees could get all the asbestos insulation and roof shingles you wanted at cost."

Later, things began to go wrong. "My brother worked at the plant for only a year, but he died of mesothelioma," said Stella. "So did Joe's sister. Nearly everyone I worked with began to die."

Joe worked in the automotive pool for most of his career at J-M and thus minimized his asbestos exposure. "Almost all the guys I worked with are now long gone," he said. "The asbestos got them."

Joe and Stella were given a number of physical exams by the J-M doctors over the years, which included chest X rays. "They told me I had some plaque but told me it was no problem," Joe said "I didn't know what that was, so I didn't worry about it. I believed what they told me."

Private medical exams have since revealed that both Joe and Stella have asbestosis. Stella received workers' compensation and then filed suit against Johns-Manville. The company paid her $100,000, but the money was immediately confiscated by New Jersey state officials. "They insisted I pay them for the workers' compensation I received," said Stella. "Then they wrote me a letter urging me to sue Johns-Manville again. I guess they wanted more money."

Johns-Manville paid Joe $60,000 for his disease. "By the time my lawyer and the state took their shares, I received less than twenty thousand dollars," said Joe. "I guess that's what I got for sixty percent of my lungs being gone."

When Joe reflected on the hundreds of his colleagues and friends who became victims of the asbestos dust, he feels fortunate. "I'm eighty-two years old. I can't sing or whistle or even walk very far anymore, but I'm alive. I guess you'd call me one of the lucky ones."

Bill and Alice Poch were not as lucky. Bill became chronically ill when he was in his mid-forties, and by age fifty he coughed constantly and struggled to breathe. The company doctors at J-M blamed it on the pipe he sometimes smoked. Alice's sister, who also worked for J-M, got sick with similar symptoms. She did not smoke. Sometimes she and Alice talked and wondered if the ubiquitous dust at the plant had anything to do with the number of people who seemed to have chronic coughs. She died of lung disease less than a decade later.

When Bill Sr. retired at the then-mandatory age of sixty-five, he went to see a private doctor about his breathing problems. "He was diagnosed immediately with mesothelioma," said Bill Jr., who still lives in Manville. "Dad went downhill quickly after that. He suffered tremendously. He was in constant pain every time he took a breath. I've never seen anything so pathetic and terrible in my life. It was impossible for him to even have a conversation; he was so distracted by the pain. The last time I saw him before he died, he was in an oxygen tent in the hospital. Finally, his lungs just couldn't take in enough air to keep him alive."

The company paid Alice $180 per month for her husband's death. She also received retirement benefits of less than $100. In 1981, Alice died of asbestosis.

Today, few people in Manville like to talk about the past. "Nearly all the people here who would complain or bring charges against the company are dead," said Joe Utasi. "Those of us who are left are just trying to live the rest of our lives without bitterness."

The company abandoned its Manville site in 1986 but was forced to clean it up after the EPA labeled the factory area one of the most toxic sites in America. Today, few traces of the company remain in Manville. In the end, all that Johns-Manville left the city were its name and a lingering legacy of betrayal and disease.

5

FOLLOWING
THE TOXIC TRAIL

"I remember we used to take hunks of vermiculite up to my aunt's house. We'd sneak up behind her and put a match under it. It pops, you know, when it's heated, and she'd jump a mile. She'd turn and scold us: 'That stuff is going to be the death of you, yet.' It turns out she was right."

—*Jim Racicot*

The intersection between the events in Libby and the national story of asbestos begin in earnest in the 1950s, when vermiculite began being marketed around the country. The vermiculite itself was considered a miracle of nature in Libby, bounty from the earth that provided jobs, security, and a product that could be shared with the country.

For the children of the town, the shiny gold and black, puffy mineral was the best plaything around. "We played in the vermiculite piles all the time," Gayla Benefield recalled. "It was like rolling around in heaps of colored popcorn. The men would bring it home from the mine and entertain the family by lighting it up. If you got it hot, it would expand like those little 'snakes' kids have on the

Fourth of July. It was mostly a gold color and that's what it was to us—real gold. For the miners and their families, the vermiculite mine was our bread and butter."

From the 1960s through the late 1980s, the Grace Company extracted and sold more than sixteen million tons of vermiculite throughout the United States and to several countries around the world. During that time the Libby mine produced nearly 80 percent of the world's vermiculite. In its expanded form, the peculiar ore was used as loose-fill insulation, acoustical sound deadeners, and in a variety of lawn and garden products. In its crushed form, it was used in cement mixes, brake shoes and pads, fireproof safes, paints, animal feeds, fertilizer, insulation, pesticides, and in a number of building products.

Each workday at the Libby mine, Bob Wilkins supervised the dumping of hundreds of pounds of raw vermiculite, which was a blackish, slatelike mineral, into rail cars to be taken to 515 different sites throughout the United States. Most were storage areas, but there were at least thirty-three processing plants in Portland, Los Angeles, Denver, Atlanta, Detroit, Minneapolis, and other cities, according to the EPA. The vermiculite was heated and expanded, or "popped," at the processing plants, and used to form a product that Grace marketed as Zonolite Attic Insulation.

It is possible to follow a distinct trail of exposure, sickness, and death that followed the vermiculite around the country. It led from the Libby miners to the rail yard workers who unloaded the vermiculite to the employees of the processing plants and finally to potentially millions of American homeowners and consumers who are still being exposed to it today.

"Nobody knows for sure how many homes in America still have Zonolite in their attics," said Dan Thornton, an EPA environmental scientist in Washington, D.C., and part of a team that attempted to retrace the trail of vermiculite. "There are no records anywhere that can help us find out which houses have it. We asked Grace and they could only say that the number of houses with Zonolite in them was 'in the millions.' We can't possibly track them down because of the lack of data."

Grace executives still deny that Zonolite, which they stopped manufacturing in the 1980s, is dangerous William Corcoran, Grace's vice president of public affairs, wrote to EPA administrator Christine Whitman in April 2002. ". . . There is no credible reason to believe [Zonolite] has ever caused an asbestos-related disease in anyone who has used it in his/her home," Corcoran wrote. He said company scientists found the insulation contains "biologically in-significant amounts" of asbestos fibers.

Health officials disagree. Assistant Surgeon General Hugh Sloan of the U.S. Public Health Service issued a warning that the in-sulation posed a "substantial health risk" to those who encounter it. Other officials advise against disturbing the vermiculite in any way. This warning gives a chilling edge to the fact that the fireproofing spray used in the bottom forty to seventy-nine floors of the North Tower of the World Trade Center was made with Libby vermiculite, according to Dr. Thomas Cahill, a University of California at Davis expert on atmospheric sciences. Dr. Cahill worked on-site at Ground Zero immediately following the terrorists' attack.

When the EPA began to follow the trail to the vermiculite ex-panding plants around the country in 2000, the agency found that most of them remained highly polluted with tremolite asbestos fibers. In some instances, the plants had closed down and new busi-nesses took over the sites without any knowledge of the danger.

Doctors, lawyers, and family members of former workers at a vermiculite processing plant in Minneapolis are blaming the as-bestos dust from the plants for the deaths of former workers and area residents. The plant, which was located on several parcels of land, processed vermiculite from Libby from 1936 until 1989. Besides the typical exposure pathways that workers and consumers faced, children often played in the waste material, called stoner rock, near the processing centers. The stoner rock, which was given away free to be used as fill or base material, contained between 2 and 10 percent tremolite asbestos. Not only were the processing plants highly contaminated, but the EPA found that dozens of nearby properties were also covered with dangerous amounts of asbestos. The government is currently working on cleaning up the sites.

Some of the other more polluted sites were in Hamilton Township, New Jersey; New Castle, Pennsylvania; Newport, Kentucky; Denver, Colorado; Minot, North Dakota; Newark, California; Los Angeles, California; Phoenix, Arizona; Portland, Oregon; and Spokane, Washington. Nearly all the other sites tested had some level of asbestos contamination. Many of them were located in heavily trafficked industrial areas and some were near residential neighborhoods. Most of the cleanup has been at the expense of American taxpayers via the EPA and other federal and state agencies.

Because of the latency period attendant to asbestos fibers, the health problems caused nationwide by the Libby vermiculite are only now being fully realized. "We used to bag that stuff with our hands. Nobody ever said anything about the fact that it might be dangerous," said John Dorsey, who worked in a Zonolite Insulation plant in Newark, California, from 1968 through 1972. "After it was mixed, we shoved the Zonolite into fifty-pound bags as fast as we could," he recalled. "We were expected to fill fifteen pallets per person per shift. It was hard, dusty work."

The Zonolite at Newark, an East San Francisco Bay suburb, was made from a mix of gypsum, vermiculite from Libby, and chrysotile asbestos. "The vermiculite was first sent through a hopper where it was heated so it would expand," said Dorsey. "Then they would take a bag of gypsum, which was a soapy-like material, and mix it with the vermiculite and raw asbestos. The asbestos would come in bricks, wrapped in paper. We'd have to pick it up with our hands and drop it in the mixer. It would all drop through a chute and get mixed again. You wouldn't believe how dusty the whole process was."

The asbestos bricks arrived in railroad cars. "The asbestos was packed like ground coffee," Dorsey said. "Once you split open the sack, it would just fall apart and you'd have to scoop it up."

Dorsey never saw warning signs at the plant. "I was covered in dust every day," he said. "The asbestos was whitish-gray and my hair was pure white after work. We never wore any protective gear, except the little paper masks they gave us. We didn't even wear gloves. The sacks went out on trucks and said 'Zonolite' on the side. I never saw anything on those sacks that said there was asbestos inside."

Dorsey, who was twenty years old when he first began working at the plant, was meticulous by nature. He made it a point to shower and change clothes before returning home. "I know now that by doing that I reduced the levels of exposure to my wife, but she washed my work clothes," he said. "She hasn't shown signs of the disease, but I still worry about her."

There were two shifts at the Newark plant with a minimum of ten people on each shift. Dorsey has not kept in touch with any of the other workers so he doesn't know how many others have been affected. "I do remember that we all liked our jobs well enough," he said. "We were making four dollars an hour, which seemed like a lot at the time. None of us had any problem with the management of the plant. Of course, now we know they weren't telling us one little secret."

In the late 1990s, Dorsey's health began to decline. He coughed frequently and often felt short of breath. His older brother, who suffered from the same symptoms, had worked in an asbestos pipe factory in San Jose and had already been diagnosed with asbestosis. By 2001, Dorsey's condition had worsened and his brother suggested that he see a physician. He was diagnosed with an advanced case of asbestosis.

Dorsey believes that the disease was caused by his handling of the sacks of chrysotile asbestos. It wasn't until the spring of 2002 that he learned of the tremolite contamination in the vermiculite. "I had no idea I was being exposed to two types of asbestos," he said. "All that dust and no warnings—that's a hell of a thing to do to somebody . . . a hell of a thing."

Over the years, the vermiculite in Libby literally became part of the town. Earl Lovick and the other mine executives allowed residents inexpensive and often free use of the expanded vermiculite. Residents took it by the pickup load to use as home insulation and in their gardens as soil conditioner. They crammed the loose-fill insulation into attics, behind walls, and under floorboards. They often sent the smallest children in the family into the tight attic spaces to pack in the vermiculite insulation. It was a rare home in Libby that wasn't filled with the golden kernels of vermiculite, which were the size and shape of a pencil eraser.

"I thought that Grace was being mighty magnanimous by letting everyone in town have as much of it as they liked," said Bob Wilkins. "It didn't even matter if you worked at the mine. You were welcome to it, tremolite and all."

Today, the estimated cost of the health screening of the residents and the cleanup of the vermiculite from the homes, gardens, garages, and lawns in Libby is about $110 million, according to the EPA. "Free, contaminated vermiculite—quite a gesture on Grace's part, wasn't it?" said Wilkins. "It only cost a hundred and ten million dollars and hundreds of people their lives. Now that's a hell of a deal."

Vermiculite is the mineralogical name given to hydrated laminar magnesium-aluminum-iron silicate, which can be found in Colorado, South Carolina, and Montana, and in Russia, Brazil, and South Africa. In its pure form, vermiculite is not dangerous. "The problem is that vermiculite is rarely pure, it is usually a very dirty ore," said Thornton. "You usually find a vein with about ten percent vermiculite and about ninety percent other materials. But, in Libby, it was different. It appears the area was once part of a super-volcano that cooked the area under extreme pressure."

Unlike most other deposits, the Libby vermiculite was formed quickly in huge sheets, leaving a vast deposit of the blackish-brown, shiny mineral that capped an entire mountainside. It would have been a seemingly endless supply of useable ore except for the fact that the same geologic forces that created the vermiculite also formed giant blocks of tremolite. The two minerals become intertwined to such a degree that it is extremely difficult, if not impossible, to separate them. Geologists and the EPA were shocked at the huge amounts of the fibrous tremolite that covered the mountain. "We have pictures of EPA inspectors in HazMat suits climbing on tremolite boulders the size of school buses," said Thornton. "It is exceedingly rare to have that type of geologic structure."

It was prospectors in search of gold and silver who first threw up a tent-and-clapboard town and called it Libby Creek after a miner's daughter in the late 1800s. When the little mining town burned to the ground before the turn of the century, it was moved to its present site near the Kootenai River and the name was shortened to

Libby. When the railroad came through and the Libby Lumber and Development Company constructed the sawmill, the isolated Montana town took on a feeling of permanency.

Perhaps no individual was more important to Libby's past— or to its future, for that matter—than a wandering mining engineer by the name of Edward Alley. A Nebraska native, Alley, like most of the men and women who always seem to present themselves in those brief seams of time when the future bends at a right angle from the past, was an adventurer and an entrepreneur who, while searching for one thing, found another that would prove of even greater importance.

Early in 1916, just before the United States entered World War I, there was a national shortage of "war materials" such as vanadium, molybdenum, and others. Alley headed for Montana in search of rich vanadium deposits he believed lay north of Libby. During the spring of that year, Alley was examining a quartz stringer in an old mine cut by silver prospectors thirty-five years before. It was pitch-black in the mine and Alley lit a burning torch. He hadn't walked far into the mine shaft when he heard a strange sputtering, crackling sound. He looked around to see that his torch had brushed up against the wall and, to his amazement, pieces of the heated mineral wall popped and puffed up like popcorn and floated around him. His curiosity piqued, Alley chiseled out a piece of ore from the wall, took it home, and heated it on his stove. He was astonished to see it turn a golden color and swell up to several times its original size. The pieces looked like gold nuggets, but they were light and water absorbent. Alley didn't know what he had found, but he sensed he could find a market for it.

For the next few years, Alley explored the entire mountainside and was excited to see that the shiny black rock seemed to be everywhere. The only trouble was no one to whom he showed the popped vermiculite took him seriously. They refused to believe it was a natural mineral. It was more than a year later that Alley traveled to New York and finally found investors for his fledgling company.

When Alley returned to his home on the Kootenai River, two miles north of Libby, he built a huge rock and clay furnace on his property. The first loads of ore from the mountain were heated and expanded in Alley's furnace. Soon, he was processing four tons a day.

In 1927, he commissioned a complete study of the area, which he dubbed Zonolite Mountain. The study revealed that there were more than forty million tons of easily identifiable vermiculite, and perhaps far more tonnage deep under the surface. Alley's mining claim ultimately covered twelve hundred acres.

An entrepreneur at heart, Alley knew the power of marketing. He advertised his mysterious mineral heavily throughout the United States, touting it as having thirteen "magical" qualities. His brochures included the following:

1. It is absolutely non-flammable; as truly so as a piece of granite.
2. It is fireproof up to 2,462 degrees.
3. It is lighter than cork—and a substitute for cork in many uses.
4. It is vermin proof—impervious to the attacks of insects, worms, and rodents.
5. It is insoluble in water and acid.
6. It is unaffected by weather. It absorbs water, but is not affected by either the absorption or evaporation process.
7. It is equal to mica as a dielectric—in other words, there is no better electric insulation substance now in commercial use.
8. It is impervious to heat or cold.
9. It is very effective as a sound deadener.
10. It is unequalled as a decorative feature.

11. It is highly adaptable to dozens of commercial uses.

12. It is a low-cost binding agent.

13. It is cheap.

By the 1930s, Alley's big dreams were coming true. The mine was paying off grandly as his company was exporting Zonolite throughout the United States, Canada, England, Belgium, Japan, and China. It was used widely to enhance acoustics in buildings, sound stages; in movie studios of Hollywood and elsewhere; in theaters; in agricultural products for everything from animal feed to fertilizer; in scores of construction and industrial products; and later in nuclear waste disposal sites and in new fireplaces nationwide as decorative embers.

The gushing writers of the day took to calling vermiculite "Montana's Marvel." None of them carried the story, though, a few decades later, when the handsome, dashing Alley was reduced to a bent and sickly man who died a hard, coughing death of "fibrosis." He was, perhaps, Zonolite Mountain's first victim.

In 1963, the year it acquired the Zonolite mine, Grace was already one of the world's leading specialty chemical companies. Nine years before, Peter Grace had orchestrated the purchase of the Davison Chemical and the Dewey & Almy Chemical companies, establishing the basis for new markets in plastic packaging, silicas, and a number of construction product lines and automobile brake parts that included asbestos ingredients. In 1958, Grace built the Washington Research Center, a large industrial-chemicals research center in Maryland. During the next two years, it also opened offices in Mexico, Venezuela, and Japan. In the 1960s, the company pioneered breakthrough methods of waterproofing homes and in petroleum catalysts that allowed refineries to increase output. As one of the fastest-growing companies in the world, it expanded its food packaging and other plants in the United Kingdom, France, Germany, Italy, Hong Kong, the Philippines, and Australia.

By 1970, when Grace introduced what would ultimately become its most controversial product, it was a powerful company led by a powerful president who had international clout. Peter Grace was easily able to pull the strings within the U.S. regulatory agencies that allowed his company to reap huge profits from an asbestos spray-on fireproofing material called Monokote.

When the story of the asbestos-contaminated Monokote finally broke in the *New York Times* in July 2001, it came as a shock to New Yorkers and to the rest of America. But, to the people of Libby, there was a collective shrug. "What else did you expect?" said Bob Wilkins. "Grace did to New York what it had been doing to Libby for years. People there are just finding out how that company operated all those years. We've known it for some time now."

The original Zonolite Company in Libby made the first versions of Monokote. The spray, which contained high amounts—at least 12 percent—of asbestos in the 1960s, was used on schools, hotels, commercial buildings, and some homes throughout America. When Grace bought the company in 1963, they continued the production of Monokote, calling their upgraded line Monokote 5.

In 1973, the fledgling EPA, which had been created just three years earlier, placed a ban on the spray application of asbestos-containing materials. Appropriately, the ban went into effect on July 4. But Grace officials took the lead in lobbying hard for an asbestos threshold level that would allow Monokote to stay on the market. In the end, the regulatory agencies bent to industry pressure. Products that contained less than 1 percent asbestos were to be exempted from the EPA's and OSHA's rules; officially, they were considered to contain no asbestos at all. The 1-percent threshold came to be known as the Grace Rule. Reflecting the industry-engineered state of many of the federal government's asbestos regulations, the Grace Rule remains the standard today.

Buoyed by its success, Grace went to war on all fronts for Monokote. When the federal government attempted to lower worker-safety standards beyond Grace's liking, the company threw up a multitude of legal barriers that tied up the regulators in court for years, effectively halting government enforcement of the rules. Meanwhile, Grace eliminated the chrysotile asbestos from the product and seized the opportunity to loudly advertise that due to a "research breakthrough," Monokote was now "asbestos-free." In the 1970s, environmental awareness was sweeping the country and the marketing ploy allowed Grace to get a serious jump on its competitors. Monokote went from just another product to the market leader in a short period of time.

What Grace had done, according to the *Times*, was replace the chrysotile asbestos in Monokote with crushed vermiculite from the Libby mine, which was, of course, contaminated with tremolite. Grace would later argue that the expanding process greatly reduced the tremolite content. While that was true, some of the deadly tremolite remained in the product. Moreover, what Grace failed to add was that the tremolite fibers that were "lost" during the expanding process polluted not only the town of Libby but the vermiculite expanding plants located around the country.

The *Times* article, written by Michael Moss and Adrianne Appel, chronicled the Grace cover-up in detail. It revealed that in 1977, Grace officials huddled at company offices in Cambridge, Massachusetts, to determine whether or not to tell the government and the consumers about the "tremolite problem" in Monokote.

"There, documents show, they weighed the risks and stayed the course," the *Times* article disclosed. "While silence increased the danger of being sued, they calculated, disclosure could have meant the end of Monokote. So, they decided, customers who inquired if Monokote contained asbestos were to be told that it did not."

At the same time, the company campaigned hard against applying hazard warning labels on Monokote and its other products. In an eighteen-page intracompany memo that outlined the company's strategy for dealing with the "tremolite problem," Grace executive vice president Elwood S. Wood stated: "The risk of liability to customers is heightened by the decision not to label our products. Based on advice of corporate counsel, this risk is categorized as moderate. . . . We believe that a decision to affix asbestos warning labels to our products would result in substantial sales losses."

By 1977, Monokote was America's top-selling fireproofing product. Grace estimated that it was used on 60 to 80 percent of the roughly 150,000 steel-frame structures built during the 1970s and 1980s. At least one expert, Dr. David Egilman, clinical associate professor at the Department of Community Health at Brown University, estimated that more than two hundred thousand pounds of pure asbestos fiber from Grace were used in the World Trade Center.

By 1980, Grace had achieved its goal—market domination and maximum profits from Monokote. They had used the strategy of minimal disclosure, first pioneered by Johns-Manville and Raybestos-Manhattan, with great success. Other companies, including the United States Mineral Products Company, were beginning to move on Monokote, though. USMP had truly replaced the asbestos in their product with a mineral wool. In trade magazine advertisements, USMP began challenging Grace to certify their materials as being free from asbestos.

Grace executives huddled up again, this time weighing a decision on whether or not to place an "asbestos" label on Monokote to cut down on potential legal suits from consumers and applicators. Peter Grace chose a tortuous course of partial disclosure, designed to ease the company's culpability with the government while continuing to hide the tremolite contamination from customers.

Part of the reason Grace had such maneuvering room was that in the 1970s and 1980s—much like today—the different regulatory agencies had sliding threshold levels for workplace and product asbestos levels. Moreover—much like today—there was no uniform method among governmental agencies to measure asbestos exposure. At that time, the EPA measured asbestos by weight, while OSHA measured it by fibers in the air. OSHA was considering lowering its limit to one hundred thousand fibers per cubic meter, considered hazardously high today by many experts. But, as the *Times* reported: "Under pressure from Grace and other companies, [OSHA] instead adopted a five million f/cm limit and lowered it only gradually . . ."

This arbitrary setting of standards reflected the success of the asbestos industry's minimal disclosure strategy. It also underscores why the tragic events in Libby are so critical. Despite current efforts by Grace to downplay the amount of sickness due to exposure there, Libby remains vital to our understanding of the extent to which asbestos can devastate human health.

Grace showed its hand as part of the effort to conceal the dangers in 1976 when it hired a researcher, William E. Smith, to inject hamsters with tremolite from Libby. One in ten developed tumors. "Then, Dr. Smith suggested injecting a fresh group with smaller amounts to test Grace's assertion that a safe level could be found," the *Times* reporters wrote. Grace rejected his proposal, interviews and documents show. " 'I guess they felt they had the answer,' said Dr. Smith, now retired. 'The material was carcinogenic.' "

At the same time, Grace's independent laboratory studies

showed that some Monokote samples contained as much as 5 percent tremolite asbestos. Other samples had very little due to the unpredictable nature of the tremolite intrusions into the vermiculite.

Today, Grace markets an asbestos-free version of Monokote, but the company maintains that their older, tremolite-containing products were safe. In a press release issued in August of 2000, the company, while no longer calling Monokote "asbestos-free," insists that it was a safe product. "Grace & Co. reaffirmed that its Monokote 4 and Monokote 5 fireproofing products sold in the U.S. from 1970 to 1989 contained trace amounts of naturally occurring asbestos . . . ," the release stated. "We believe these products were safe when they were installed and are safe in place today," said Paul J. Norris, current Grace chairman, president, and CEO. "It was well-known to regulatory agencies and many of our customers that minute quantities of naturally occurring asbestos were in our products. We are making this announcement to make sure that everyone hears the facts from Grace."

The attempted "spin" in the release can be seen in the carefully chosen description of "trace amounts of naturally occurring asbestos," which almost seems like the description of a breakfast cereal that is good for your heart. What they left out, of course, is that even trace amounts of this "naturally occurring" ingredient can kill a human in some of the most inhumane ways possible. It also indicates that the vermiculite is "safe in place," meaning that as long as it is not disturbed it will not harm the occupants. That ignores, of course, the likelihood that at some point homeowners or professional electricians, plumbers, etc., will disturb the insulation while remodeling or maintaining the house.

The press release did end with a series of facts that Grace has always been quick to reveal. It boasted that Grace has "annual sales of approximately $1.5 billion, over 6,000 employees and operations

in nearly 40 countries." Monokote sales played a major role in creating the robust health of the company.

The first tremors that foreshadowed problems within Grace's empire came in the late 1970s in the unlikely town of Marysville, Ohio.
Like Libby, Marysville was a sleepy, rural community in the 1970s
and 1980s, supported economically by a large industrial plant just
outside of town. Marysville, which is about twenty miles northwest
of Columbus, is the home of the nation's largest producer of do-it-
yourself lawn and garden products, the Scotts Company. The company, then known as O. M. Scotts and Sons, opened the Marysville
factory in 1957 and began making and marketing lawn and garden
fertilizers, pesticides, and herbicides. During that time, company scientists found an unusual material that supported all these products
in a number of ways, including as a water carrier and soil conditioner. The product was vermiculite, and the source was Libby.

"Scott was by far the biggest customer of vermiculite from
Libby," said Dan Thornton, whose team processed more than fifty-
six thousand invoices taken from Grace's mine headquarters in
Libby. "Scott used about 523,000 tons of Libby vermiculite over the
years." (A processing plant in Santa Ana, California, was the next
biggest user, with a total of 425,000 tons.)

The story that unfolded at Marysville is eerily similar to the
story of Manville and Libby and the other blue-collar towns around
the world that have had the misfortune to be involved with asbestos. According to a series of investigative stories by *Columbus
Dispatch* environmental reporter Michael Hawthorne, Scotts's executives were told by Grace in 1971 that its vermiculite was contaminated with tremolite. Even though that warning was followed
by an OSHA study in 1977 that found lung abnormalities in the

X rays of thirty-two Scotts employees in Marysville—one out of
every four tested—Scotts did not stop accepting vermiculite from
Libby until 1980.

"A handful of people knew about the dangers twenty-five years
ago and didn't bother sharing the information with anybody," said
Hawthorne. "The risks were always downplayed by Scotts. They will
tell you that they wet the vermiculite so there was little risk of respiratory problems. They've been playing semantic games for thirty
years."

The contaminated Scotts lawn products were shipped to millions of homes around the United States, according to Thornton.
The EPA, in 2001, also found old sacks of Scotts potting soil containing Libby vermiculite still on the shelves of a few garden stores.
Thornton downplayed the dangers to consumers, however. "It is
used primarily outdoors and it is stable for the most part, in the
lawns. It is also wet most of the time. I don't believe we are going to
see significant levels of sickness caused by those lawn products." Neither Thornton nor any other scientist can define what "significant
levels" are, however. Due to the underreporting of asbestos-related
diseases and their long latency periods, it is difficult to make that determination. Victims and physicians are still generally unaware that
the vermiculite can cause asbestos-related diseases. Often, when
mesothelioma and asbestosis victims have had no known asbestos
exposure pathways, household products or brake shoes have been
blamed.

What is known is that at least one-fourth of the Scotts workforce was sickened by the vermiculite contamination and at least five
people have died of asbestosis. These numbers are most likely conservative, according to Hawthorne.

"It is a privately held company, and it is difficult to determine
just how many people are sick," he said. "You have a medical com-

munity here that doesn't really seem to be interested in finding out about this. You have to understand that for years, Scotts ran this town. One former employee got sick and company doctors said the spots on his X rays were fatty deposits. He suspected something else, though. Before he died, he made his wife promise she would have an autopsy done. It showed that the spots weren't fat deposits but asbestos plugs."

According to reports from the *Columbus Dispatch*, Scotts informed workers at the Marysville plant in 1976 that "very small traces" of asbestos had been found in the vermiculite. In 1978, a National Institute for Occupational Safety and Health (NIOSH) study found twelve cases of lung disease among Scotts workers that were attributed directly to "tremolite exposure."

In 1980, a draft of an EPA report concluded that "asbestos-contaminated vermiculite may pose a serious and widespread hazard to workers." A final version of the report was never released. That year Scotts finally reacted to the information and switched to using vermiculite from two mines in South Carolina, one owned by Virginia Vermiculite and the other by Grace. The mine operators insisted their ore was clean, but government studies show that both mines also produced asbestos-contaminated vermiculite. A twenty-four-year-old study done by the Mount Sinai School of Medicine found asbestos levels of from 2 percent to 56 percent in Virginia ore samples, according to *Dispatch* reports.

"The problem with vermiculite is the geologic conditions that allow it to form are also the same geologic conditions that allow [asbestos minerals] to form," said Al Bush, a world-renowned vermiculite expert working with the EPA in Denver. "These conditions exist almost everywhere in the world, so that asbestiform minerals and vermiculite almost always invade each other. You can take vermiculite samples at several different sites and not get the same makeups in any of them," said Bush. "The only thing we know for sure is the people in Libby are dying."

The NIOSH study done in 1978 at the Scotts plant ultimately led government researchers back to Libby. They strongly suspected that Libby vermiculite workers were going to suffer the same health problems as they saw in Ohio. Later studies confirmed their suspicions, but getting word of the dangers to the miners at Libby proved to be an unconscionably long and haphazard process.

Bob Wilkins still recalls the cool, spring day in the latter part of March 1979 when he first learned that asbestos was a danger at the mine. He was working at the railroad loading facility in Libby and had gotten to know a trim, gray-haired inspector from NIOSH named Robert Smith. Smith and a small team of scientists had followed the trail of vermiculite from the Scotts plant, but they kept a low profile, and the Libby miners thought of it as just another routine inspection. Smith seemed like a "good guy" to Wilkins. The miners agreed to wear the odd-looking monitors Smith gave them, even though Wilkins thought it was a useless exercise. The men had been reassured by Lovick that the ubiquitous dust was just a nuisance. Why bother monitoring it?

That day the government man told Wilkins that he had been all over the country doing various mineral studies. He mentioned offhandedly that he had once found a deposit of asbestos in a copper mine in Arizona.

"I'm glad we don't have any asbestos around here," Wilkins told Smith. "All we have up here in Libby is tremolite." Smith gave Wilkins a long, funny look. Without a word, he turned and walked back to his government truck. A few minutes later he came back with a huge book on rocks and minerals. He leafed through the book, finally pinning down a section with his finger, holding the page against the hardening wind.

"Look," Smith said. Wilkins leaned over and read the first sentence. "Tremolite," the book stated, "is the most dangerous form of asbestos."

Wilkins was stunned. He remembered that he had heard Lovick use the word "tremolite" from time to time as if it were some type of waste ore that was just part of the dust. He stared at Smith as his shock gave way to anger. Without saying a word, he stalked down to his truck and drove straight to Lovick's office.

Lovick was a tall, distinguished-looking man with an easy, convincing, talkative style. Wilkins later would say that Lovick "could sell an Eskimo a refrigerator." When Wilkins barged in, Lovick was sitting behind his big desk talking to the general manager of the mill, Bill McCaig. Both men were in suits. They looked up, startled, as Wilkins strode in, covered in dust.

"Earl, we've got a problem," Wilkins said angrily.

"What's the matter?" Lovick asked. "Your union got a gripe?"

"Yeah, we've got a gripe all right," Wilkins said. "For years, you've been telling us that dust is just a nuisance dust. Why the hell didn't you tell us that tremolite is asbestos?"

Lovick spread his arms and shrugged. "Hell, Bob, I thought everybody knew that."

Wilkins couldn't believe what Lovick was saying. "You know they don't," he said. "There isn't a man up there on that hill who knows what tremolite is. But you can bet your ass they are all going to know at the next union meeting."

During the next few years, the vermiculite miners in Libby were surveyed, studied, analyzed, and written about by a variety of government scientists. Papers with titles like "The Morbidity and Mortality of Vermiculite Miners and Millers Exposed to Tremolite-Actinolite: Part III. Radiographic Findings" were printed in the *American Journal of Industrial Medicine*. The increased rates of lung abnormalities in the Libby miners were evaluated and categorized with some regularity. The dust at the mine and the asbestos content were found to be out of compliance with state and federal rules in nearly every inspection, despite the fact that the mine was nearly always tipped off to the inspections three days in advance. At the same time, Wilkins kept his word and told the men about the tremolite dangers.

Yet from 1980 to 1990, very little changed at the mine. The EPA has since admitted that it "dropped the ball" when it came to enforcing the regulations that Grace ignored with such frequency. An Office of the Inspector General's report released March 31, 2001, stated, "Although EPA made attempts to address contaminant asbestos exposure like that in Libby, those attempts did not result in regulations or other controls that might have protected the citizens of Libby."

The OIG report assigned much of the blame on poor intra-agency communication and budget constraints. It skirted around what insiders feel was the real reason the EPA failed to do its duty— the close friendship between President Ronald Reagan and Peter Grace.

"The revelations at the Scotts plant in 1979 caused the government to look at Libby," said a source within the EPA. "If you look at the correspondence back then, the memos and reports are almost strident about the disease capabilities of vermiculite. In 1979–80, the EPA developed a rather elaborate plan to look at vermiculite processing centers around the country. We actually started doing some of these investigations when they were suddenly stopped. The principle leader of these investigations said someone came into his office a month after Reagan took office and said, 'Stop working on this. It isn't a priority anymore.' It was that linear."

Not long afterward, Reagan appointed Peter Grace to head up one of the most powerful commissions in the country. His mission was to find ways of stripping away government regulations.

"The OIG report says it was the lack of communications," added the EPA source. "But, the truth is, it was a case where the administration just wasn't interested in pursuing the health effects of vermiculite. They chose profits over lives; it was a clear-cut choice."

The OIG report also found a number of grievous errors made by the EPA staff. There were lost documents and unexplained lack of enforcement actions against Grace. A 1980 memo showed that someone in the EPA made the critical judgment that vermiculite did not merit government regulation. Had the reverse been true, the EPA would have "fast-tracked" an analysis to determine whether to fully investigate the health risks in Libby and elsewhere. The memo was written despite the findings at the Scotts plant. Later, according to the OIG report, the official who signed the memo "couldn't recall exactly why EPA determined [the enforcement section] did not apply."

Perhaps most grievous of all was this paragraph from the OIG report:

In August, 1982, EPA completed a draft disposition paper regarding asbestos-contaminated vermiculite. The paper concluded that there were significant adverse health effects associated with past occupational exposure probably caused by inhalation of the asbestos that contaminated the vermiculite. The paper also stated that the public was generally unaware that vermiculite was likely to be contaminated with asbestos. In addition, it stated that there was no regulatory control of consumer use, and some consumer uses may pose a significant health hazard. It proposed recommendations that governmental agencies test the vermiculite and measure the level of consumer exposure to asbestos in selected vermiculite products. EPA officials were unable to find a final version of the disposition paper, which was never released.

Had this report been acted upon in 1982, it could potentially have saved hundreds and perhaps even thousands of people in Libby and the surrounding communities—including all the Little Leaguers who played on Libby's contaminated baseball fields until 1998. It would have also prevented perhaps millions of consumers across the country from being exposed to Zonolite products. The mysterious disappearance of the draft report has never been explained.

It was clear that although the miners had been told about the tremolite, few, if any, knew the real dangers it presented. "I think they knew there was some type of a problem," said Libby resident Jim Racicot. "But up here in Libby you either went into the military, worked at the sawmill or at the mine. Each choice had its risks and you just had to be cowboy-tough about it. The attitude here has always been you take whatever hand is dealt to you and you don't complain. The working men in Libby didn't have much say-so over their economic lives, but they could be a hero to their families by sticking to their jobs so there was food on the table, even if it meant risking their health. They just didn't know that the tremolite would put their families in jeopardy as well."

The suffering caused by asbestos among these everyday working heroes and their families cannot be summed up in a graph or in a neat table of statistics. The masses that grew around the asbestos fibers in former Scotts worker Lloyd Gordon's lungs were so great that before he died, doctors, in desperation, peeled his lungs like an orange. Even after the surgery he was in constant pain and coughed up round, hard balls of tissue and fiber. His skin was gray, a telltale sign of who has asbestosis in Marysville. The victims' skin usually turned the color of iron, and they moved slowly on the sidewalks, stopping frequently to catch their breath.

Gordon wasn't always that way. Once he was robust, full of energy and love for his young daughter. "I was nineteen when my dad died," said his daughter, Linda Schwendenman. "It was sixteen years ago and I still have a lot of anger . . . just talking about it again I won't sleep for a week. I want him back. I feel cheated."

No one ever told Gordon that there was asbestos hidden inside the vermiculite that he ran through the heat-expander every workday at the Scotts Company plant for ten years. He didn't mind the job, but he lived for the weekends, when he would practice his photography and craft silver jewelry for friends. He took tons of pictures of Linda and made her little bits of jewelry as she got older. He was a carpet installer by trade, but when the job at Scotts opened up in the late 1960s, Gordon took it. Health insurance became a priority when Linda was born, and Scotts had a good health plan.

"He took that job because of me," said Schwendenman. "I feel guilty to this day about that. He did what a good father would do and it killed him."

Linda's mother, Alice, remembered her husband as vibrant and even tempered. "I remember the last time he was healthy," she said. "It was in 1976. He had just been promoted, and his boss complimented him for being so honest and always being on time for work. He was making more than eight dollars an hour then, and we had just gotten to where we could save a little."

In 1977, when Gordon was thirty-nine years old, he had a heart attack. Later, doctors would attribute his heart problems to the lack of oxygen caused by the asbestosis, but at the time they blamed it on his cigarettes. He stopped smoking, recovered, and went back to work. The company made him take a different job and reduced his pay to five dollars an hour. Gordon never fully recovered his health. He began to cough incessantly, and he always seemed to be suffering from colds and other respiratory diseases.

By the early winter of 1977, Gordon was too sick to work. For the next nine years he lived in constant pain, his health slowly deteriorating. "It was so hard to watch," said Alice. "He got old before our eyes. When he was in his forties, he looked like he was seventy."

Gordon's life became a series of trips to various hospitals. He was given several different diagnoses before his lungs began to fill with fluid and collapsed. He was finally diagnosed with asbestos-related pulmonary failure at the University of Kentucky Chandler Medical Center. For the first time, the Gordons began to believe it was the asbestos exposure Lloyd suffered at his job at the Scotts plant that was killing him.

"I felt right then that the Scotts people knew about this all along and didn't tell us," Alice said. "I was so mad that if I was a bomber I would have blown that plant up. I just don't know how to make a bomb."

Gordon died in 1986. No representative from Scotts attended the funeral. "I don't know how to get past my anger and frustration," said Schwendenman. "What can you do when your father dies needlessly because people wanted a bigger profit? They've never been held accountable for what they did."

Alice misses her husband every day. "We had a good relationship and a good life," she said. "I don't want to cry, but parts of it you never get over. I just think that money goes a long way in this country in deciding who is going to live and who is going to die."

6

1940–1980:
THE COVER-UP

In the twentieth century, America consumed more than thirty million metric tons of asbestos, more than two-thirds of it after WWII. The years between 1940 and 1980 were boom times for the asbestos industry. By the time they were over, asbestos could be found in nearly every automobile, airplane, attic, appliance, building, bus, truck, and train in America, despite public knowledge of its dangers. Much of it remains there today.

During those four decades, the industry grew into a multibillion-dollar enterprise that employed more than two hundred thousand people, according to the Travelers' Insurance Company, which insured Johns-Manville and several other companies.

They were also decades of a deepening and ever-more successful corporate cover-up of the dangers of asbestos products. This occurred in spite of the emergence of an outspoken critic of the industry, Dr. Irving Selikoff, the charismatic director of the Environmental Sciences Laboratory at the Mount Sinai Hospital in New York City.

Monitoring and enforcement of air-quality laws by government regulators could have reduced the exposure that so many workers suffered, but the postwar years were defined by a deep fear and hatred of communism and an abiding belief in the sacredness of American corporations. Governmental meddling in the realm of free enterprise was met with an immediate red flag. *Laissez-aller* was the governmental attitude toward big business, and in the twenty-five years following WWII, an unfettered corporate America spun out profits and pollution in record amounts.

Yet even during these boom times, the leaders of the asbestos industry, made arrogant by their success, were making decisions that would ultimately sow the seeds of their companies' financial destruction.

No one personified that arrogance more than Lewis Brown, president of Johns-Manville, which, by 1940, had become a world leader in asbestos product sales.

On June 4, 1940, a "Lewis H. Brown Dinner" was held in the Kansas City Club in Kansas City, Missouri, to honor the Johns-Manville president. Many of the powerful, conservative businessmen and politicians in the Midwest attended.

The keynote speech that night was given by J. C. Nichols, a wealthy Kansas City real estate developer. Nichols's fiery speech concentrated on the growing public debt and the increase in the cost of government. "With all this rapid increase, how long can free enterprise continue?" he railed, echoing Brown's often-repeated sentiments. "How long will any individual strive to earn? How long will our democracy survive? Soon—very soon—will there be any real difference between Hitler's, Stalin's, and Mussolini's way of life and our own American way of living unless some check can be made in our mad, unthinking race to ruin—in our reckless waste of not only the earnings of our enslaved people, but the possible nationalization of business and industry and ultimate confiscation of property itself? Will entrenched bureaucrats become masters of us all?"

Nichols's speech was met with a thunderous ovation, and most likely nobody applauded harder than Brown himself. An Iowa University graduate and an army veteran, Brown was then forty-six years old, a grandfather, chairman of the Red Cross in New York, and president of a company that employed twelve thousand people in seventeen plants around the country and in Canada. He was one of the most powerful industrialists in the world.

Brown was outspoken in his hatred for communism and his belief that big business represented what was right in America. In 1943, he founded the American Enterprise Institute (AEI), a non-profit organization that he envisioned would allow him to match the influence that Robert Somers Brookings achieved through the Brookings Institute. Brown founded AEI to be not only an intellectual counterweight to President Roosevelt's New Deal philosophies but also an active promoter of his vision of a corporate America free of all governmental restrictions and regulations. Through publications, seminars, and some political involvement, AEI was fiercely pro-military and anticommunist. One observer called AEI during Brown's era "a pro-corporation lunatic fringe."

His opposition to Soviet-style communism may have been well based, and well supported throughout the country, but it failed badly as a defensible rationalization for his callous disregard for his employees. In the years to come, an avalanche of memos, reports, and letters would surface that would give definition to just how deep his desire for profits and his distain for his workers ran.

For example, in 1949, an area physician, Dr. Kenneth Smith, sent a memo to J-M headquarters regarding seven asbestos mill employees whose X rays exhibited the beginning signs of asbestosis. Dr. Smith's memo advised Johns-Manville executives not to share the information with the workers. He wrote: "As long as the man is not disabled it is felt that he should not be told of his condition so that he can live and work in peace and the company can benefit by his many years of experience."

Brown not only accepted Dr. Smith's advice to conceal the information, he later hired him to be a medical director for Johns-Manville.

Lewis Brown's influence was felt beyond America's borders. The U.S.-owned Canadian Johns-Manville Company owned much of Quebec's "fiber belt" asbestos mines, and it was there that Lewis Brown's worst labor fears were realized. Canada's National Federation of Mining Industry Employees went out on strike in 1949, after a two-month negotiation with J-M failed. The strike closed down most of J-M's Canadian mines, including J-M's huge mining operation near the town of Asbestos, Quebec. The union had fifteen demands, including a general wage raise, but its primary concern was the asbestos dust and how it was affecting the workers and their families. When the union submitted its list of demands in writing, the first was: "The elimination of asbestos dust inside and out of the mines."

According to author Paul Brodeur, when asked during a deposition about the working conditions in the Canadian mines in the 1940s, Dr. Smith recalled what it was like. "Walking through the town of Asbestos on a dry August day, you could see little rolls of asbestos fiber rolling along the street like tumbleweed, and you just assumed that anybody walking the streets—the storekeepers, or policeman walking his beat, or anybody in the house—would be exposed to that airborne dust. And I can remember rather vividly Dr. Stevenson [whom Dr. Smith would subsequently succeed as CJ-M Medical director] . . . standing at the edge of the open pit on the eastern side. The whole town of Asbestos was behind us and, of course, the winds are constantly from the west, blowing across the mine, across the mill, and into the town. And Stevenson said, 'What a shame that the town wasn't built on that hill over there on the western side of the pit. There would have been no dust in the town.'"

Dr. Smith was then asked if anyone else heard Stevenson's statement.

"I believe A. R. Fisher was there, as I recall," said Dr. Smith. "A. R. Fisher, at that time, was the vice president, production, for the corporation in New York." (Fisher would, in 1955, become president of J-M.)

Dr. Smith was asked when the incident occurred.

"Oh, sometime between '45 and '49," he answered. "I remember that rather vividly because I picked up a piece of asbestos fiber from the rock there and was crushing it, and the chrysotile fiber—you can take the fiber and crush it with your fingers like this and make a ball of wool out of it, and in so doing I had a spicule enter my finger and later developed a small tumor there."

After the deposition, Dr. Smith provided lawyers with an industrial hygiene survey he had conducted of 708 men who worked at the mine at Asbestos. Only four had healthy lungs. Again, Dr. Smith recommended the men not be told of their condition. "Should the man be told of his condition today there is a very definite possibility that he would become mentally and physically ill, simply through the knowledge that he has asbestosis," Dr Smith wrote. He sent the report to Fisher, who sent it on to Vandiver Brown. Dr. Smith's report was not made available to the employees.

On May 5, 1949, several hundred union supporters entered the town of Asbestos and blockaded the streets so that no "scab" workers could enter the mines. They clashed with the Provincial Police, and there were a few injuries on both sides. The following day a large police force broke up the strikers, and the riot was over. The strike continued, and the miners angrily demanded dust control measures, pointing to the abnormally high rate of "tuberculosis" among the miners and their families. The strikers made great sport of the heir to the Manville fortune, Tommy Manville, who lived a colorful life but had little to do with the operations of the company. Manville ultimately got married thirteen times to eleven different women, nearly all of them blondes. Photographs of his many wives were posted around the town of Asbestos by the strikers.

Lewis Brown was infuriated by the strike, which he considered communistic in its intent. "It was apparent beyond doubt that the real issue was not wages and working conditions," a report from the headquarters at CJ-M stated. "The intent of the labor leaders was to deprive the owners of our properties of the right to use them."

Nervous that the powerful Catholic Church was backing the workers, the report attempted to appeal to the religious leaders through the liberal use of religious quotes, including this specious selection from a Papal Encyclical:

> *This error [the miners' desire for better working conditions] was much more specious than that of certain of the Social- ists who hold that whatever serves to produce goods ought to be transferred to the State, or, as they say, 'Socialized,' is consequently all the more dangerous and the more apt to deceive the unwary. It is an alluring poison which many have eagerly drunk whom open Socialism had not been able to deceive.*

Although willing to negotiate on the pay raises, CJ-M refused to discuss cleaning up the asbestos dust. In a public report, the company's official line was: "Canadian Johns-Manville Company, Ltd. has spent over $1 million to eliminate dust. Dust in the town of As- bestos is no greater than dust in the average industrial center on the continent. As a practical matter it is impossible to fulfill such an agreement as demanded."

The statement, of course, ignored all of Dr. Smith's findings that the dust, in fact, was causing disease in not only a high percentage of the miners, but many of the residents of the town of Asbestos as well.

In the end, union officials agreed to a provisional increase of ten cents an hour and reemployment of the strikers. Their new agreement with CJ-M included no mention of asbestos dust abatement.

That a few company doctors continued to betray their Hippocratic oath by withholding vital medical information from their patients is perhaps within the margins of human foibles, but in September 1952, an event occurred that cast a stain on some of the best physicians in America. Because of a collective lack of courage among them, an opportunity was lost, and the outcome would be profoundly tragic.

The Saranac Laboratories in upstate New York had long done medical experiments and studies involving asbestos, usually financed by the asbestos companies. The association dated back to 1928, when Johns-Manville sponsored research that showed that mice forced to inhale asbestos fibers suffered consequent mesothelioma and other asbestos-related diseases. The result of the test was never made public, which became standard procedure for the research done at Saranac. Most of the reports on the estimated thirteen hundred experiments done at Saranac on asbestos and other occupational diseases have mysteriously disappeared over the years.

In 1952, Saranac Laboratories nevertheless sponsored its Seventh Saranac Symposium, an ambitious event that was attended by most of the recognized asbestos experts in the world. This included federal officials, insurance company experts, and the medical directors from most of the asbestos companies. It was the first international conference ever held on asbestos. For one full week, papers were presented and talks were given on the findings of researchers and physicians around the world. Sadly, unlike the other six conferences sponsored by Saranac Laboratories, none of this information was ever published, supposedly for budgetary reasons.

Wrote Brodeur: "If a significant number of the fifty-odd medical doctors who attended the Seventh Symposium had spoken out or had insisted that its papers and discussions be made public, they might well have blown the lid off the asbestos cover-up and saved thousands of lives, untold pain and suffering, and millions of dollars. . . . Too many of them remained silent, and the conference simply marked the nadir of a year in which the asbestos industry, with the tacit approval of its insurers, successfully suppressed information about the most important industrial carcinogen the world has ever known."

There was one exception to the silence of the physicians. Dr. Wilhelm C. Hueper, chief of the environmental cancer section at the National Cancer Institute, refused to be muffled by the asbestos industry. He gave constant public warnings that not only were asbestos workers in danger from the fibers, so were those who lived by the mines and manufacturing plants. He became the first official to attempt to expose the strategy of concealment conducted by the asbestos companies. In a 1943 bulletin of the American Cancer Society, he unloaded a haymaker to the chin of the industry by saying the cover-up was an effort to avoid the expensive "technical and sanitary changes" required to protect the workers. He also accused the industry of covering up to avoid potential lawsuits. He complained bitterly when the Saranac Symposium, which he attended, was not publicized. For his efforts, he took years of abuse from the industry and their insurance companies. He was denigrated by industry "experts" and harpooned in industry literature.

In 1956, an American Mutual Liberty Company memo reflected how much the industry feared and hated Hueper. It also, co-incidentally, provided an accurate look into the future. "With a 'mad dog' like Hueper loose on the subject of asbestos, future claim results can be alarming," the memo stated.

The list of those who turned their backs on the asbestos problem extends beyond physicians. The story of Kaylo, a thermal-installation material developed by Owens-Illinois Glass Company in Ohio, is an example of the forces that conspired against asbestos workers and consumers.

Owens-Illinois, which ultimately sold the Kaylo product division to the Owens-Corning Fiberglas Company, made Kaylo from a mixture of calcium hydroxide and silica with an asbestos content of about 15 percent. It gained its name from the fact that the engineering term for the amount of heat that can pass through an inch of insulation is called the "K" factor. "Kaylo," then, boasted of the product's low heat conductivity value.

From the beginning, scientists warned the manufacturer that the product was a danger to workers. The company was warned several times throughout the 1940s, including in a 1948 letter from Saranac Laboratories published by Brodeur that stated: "In all animals sacrificed after more than 30 months exposure to Kaylo dust, unmistakable evidence of asbestosis has developed, showing that Kaylo on inhalation is capable of producing asbestosis and must be regarded as a potentially-hazardous material."

The study was followed by several others, yet Kaylo was such a hot seller that the company continued to ignore the warnings. In fact, in April 1952, E. C. Shuman, director of research at Owens-Illinois, wrote an article for *Petroleum Engineering Magazine* promoting the use of Kaylo in refineries.

"The story of how this company researched and developed the

non-glass insulating material . . . is an inspiring example of the American Way," he wrote. "Without the vision, resources, and technical know-how of 'big business,' this material would not be on the market today."

Barry Castleman has since pointed out that the photograph that accompanied the article showed an employee sawing a length of Kaylo molded pipe insulation, using a shipping carton as a bench. There is dust everywhere, and the man is not wearing a respirator.

Unfortunately for the asbestos workers, their own union proved every bit as hypocritical in the spring of 1941. When the Asbestos Workers union, in the midst of labor negotiations with Corning, threatened to claim that the company's fiberglass materials posed a health hazard, the company turned the tables by threatening to expose the health hazards of asbestos to the union's rank and file. The officials at the Asbestos Workers union, fearful that the ensuing criticism could split the union, quickly backed down from their fiberglass threat and ultimately accepted most of the company's terms.

Another nail in the workers' coffin came, incredibly, from the U.S. Public Health Service. During the 1960s, according to Brodeur's research, the chief industrial hygienist for the Health Service's Division of Occupational Health entered into a confidentiality agreement with asbestos manufacturers that prevented him from exposing details of the health dangers his inspectors encountered during their inspections of the asbestos plants. Why this mind-boggling deal was struck by a federal agency mandated to protect the public health is left to conjecture.

In Europe, as well as in much of the rest of the industrialized world, profits and disease from asbestos were on a vertical rise. The powerful English company Turner & Newall had become one of the biggest manufacturers of asbestos products in the world. By 1970, the company had a workforce of nearly thirty-seven thousand people and operated asbestos mines in Canada, Southern Rhodesia, Swaziland, and South Africa and asbestos factories in India, with subsidiaries in North America and Europe. The company's main advertising theme was that putting asbestos in skyscrapers, ships, offices, homes, theaters, and automobiles saved lives.

Workers began dying from asbestos in the English Turner & Newall plants in the 1920s. In one particularly gruesome report, Dr. Ian Grieve, who performed an autopsy on a young woman asbestos worker, noted that when her lung was cut open, "the knife almost appeared to grate," due to the massive accumulation of asbestos fibers.

The asbestos industry in South Africa covered up health dangers for decades. Typically, about one-third of all the workers in the asbestos mines were children. Some were as young as seven years old, according to a report in the *Guardian* of London. The asbestos industry there clearly knew of the dangers, but few steps were taken to protect the workers and their families.

Turner & Newall, much like its asbestos company counterparts in the United States, practiced decades of concealment. The company conducted numerous health and safety conferences, although officials saw a "danger of having too open a meeting with representatives present who were not fully familiar enough with the problem [asbestosis]," according to *Magic Mineral to Killer Dust*, a book written on the company by Geoffrey Tweedale (Oxford University Press, 2000).

"Those deemed not familiar enough with the problem included the workers and their trade unions, who were never invited to attend discussions on health," wrote Tweedale. Turner & Newall helped pay for some of the studies at the Saranac Labs but never publicized nor told its workers about the results. For their part, the

workers were aware that many of their colleagues died early of respiratory failure, but few were moved to complain. "The culture of
the textile and asbestos industries—paternalistic, deferential, and
relatively weakly unionized—obviously played a part," Tweedale
wrote.

The deadly hypocrisy that was practiced by so many American
companies was matched by Turner & Newall. Tweedale noted that
in the Christmas 1952 edition of the company's quarterly staff magazine, *Firefly*, one of Turner & Newall's longest-serving employees,
storekeeper Bill Jagger, was featured on the cover. The article on the
forty-seven-year-old Jagger did not mention that the reason Jagger
was working in the store instead of the plant was that he could not
do physical work because he was suffering from advanced cases of
asbestosis and lung cancer. The next issue carried a brief story of his
death but did not mention the cause.

In a situation that foreshadowed the tragic events yet to unfold
in Libby, Montana, Tweedale recounted the poisoning of an entire
English town by Turner & Newall's Armley factory. Included in the
exposure were many of the town's children, who played "among the
sacks of blue asbestos that [the company] had carelessly stacked outside the factory. . . . However, local residents did not complain,
fearing that family members would lose their jobs."

There were numerous public medical studies done in England
that showed exactly what the dangers were. In 1930, Dr. E. R. A.
Merewether and engineering inspector C. W. Price presented links
between asbestos and disease to Parliament, which prompted the
passage of the Asbestos Regulations in 1931. These included rules
for improved dust control and ventilation that were not imposed in
the United States for decades to come.

In 1955, Dr. Richard Doll made public his findings that the incidence of lung cancer among asbestos workers at Turner & Newall's
Rochdale plant was ten times the national norm. Other studies fol-

lowed, but Parliament, much like the American Congress, was usually slow to act on worker safety issues, when they acted at all.

It wasn't until 1964, when an international conference on asbestos convened in New York and did what the 1952 Saranac Symposium should have done, that the public received its first notice that asbestos was indeed a killer. Organized by a group headed by Dr. Irving Selikoff, the conference not only revealed asbestos as a public health hazard of terrible proportions, it propelled Dr. Selikoff to the forefront of the asbestos industry's list of enemies. Just before the conference convened, Dr. Selikoff published a report in the *Journal of the American Medical Association* that horrified asbestos company executives. During 1962–63, Dr. Selikoff, Dr. Jacob Churg, chief pathologist at the Barnert Memorial Hospital in Paterson, New Jersey, and Dr. Cuyler Hammon, an official with the American Cancer Society, conducted a study of the members of the Asbestos Workers Union in New Jersey and New York. They found that out of 392 asbestos workers who had more than twenty years of exposure, 339 had asbestosis. Among those who had died, lung cancer was found to be at least seven times more common than normal. Dr. Selikoff followed these findings with numerous other asbestos studies over the next thirty years. He wasn't the first to find that asbestos causes serious diseases, but he was outspoken, articulate, and relentless. He quickly became public enemy number one to the asbestos industry, including Turner & Newall, which he had criticized in his many studies. The company was outraged—and many medical experts were astounded—when Dr. Selikoff publicly announced that there is no "safe level" of asbestos and that even one asbestos fiber can prove lethal.

The asbestos industry's frantic fear of Dr. Selikoff surfaced in a number of intracompany memos, including this one in March 1973, written by Turner & Newall executive David Hills: "Dr. Selikoff is going off his head," wrote Hills. "We really must get onto our friends in the [American insurance industry]; this man Selikoff has got to be stopped somehow . . . he almost needs certifying."

In 1965, an Owens Corning internal memo stated: "Our present concern is to find some way of preventing Dr. Selikoff from creating problems and affecting sales."

In all, Dr. Selikoff and his medical teams studied the causes of death among 17,800 asbestos workers in the United States and Canada between 1962 and 1986. His work greatly furthered the country's understanding of the scope of the problem and remains the seminal work on asbestos done to date. In 1984, Dr. Selikoff conducted the only known medical survey of the Norfolk Naval Shipyard in Portsmouth, Virginia. Of the 142 employees whom he studied, 113 (79 percent) had lung abnormalities caused by asbestos. He also found that victims who had worked with asbestos for less than a week had scarred lungs thirty years later.

(Ironically, when the avalanche of asbestos-exposure lawsuits roared down on the judicial system in the 1980s, the asbestos industry changed tactics and tried to "canonize" Dr. Selikoff in an attempt to convince juries and judges that it wasn't until his studies in the mid-1960s that they realized asbestos was harmful.)

Dr. Selikoff's studies did cause Johns-Manville to voluntarily put mild warning labels on some of their products (much to the chagrin of many of the other asbestos companies). Yet even his strong and colorful personality and the overall weight of his work did not penetrate the consciousness of the American public. There remained little public or media outcry over the terrible conditions that continued to permeate the asbestos industry.

The asbestos industry, however, was beginning to realize its vulnerability. Workers' compensation claims were growing, and the industry feared it was just the tip of the iceberg. In the spring of 1969, a meeting of house counsel of asbestos manufacturers was held at the Johns-Manville headquarters to talk about the problem. The worried company executives talked at length about methods of handling the upcoming cases. Attending the meeting were executives of Travelers' Insurance. A ruling had just been handed down by the Workers' Compensation Board indicating a probable causal relationship between the claimant's exposure to asbestos at the workplace and his contracting cancer of the colon.

In a confidential memo dated August 12, 1969, Travelers' reported: "Doctor Selikoff's testimony was very damaging to us in this landmark case. Johns-Manville thought that this case would open the floodgates and that they as a major producer of asbestos would be in great jeopardy." The memo then shared the real fear of the insurers and the industry. "Asbestosis, lung or colon cancer claims, whether comp or liability, from asbestos workers or those working with asbestos materials, are one thing, but the general public exposure and claim potential is much more serious."

Travelers' also expressed concern over a claim brought against J-M by the executor of the estate of a Manville, New Jersey, woman named Ann Fetchko in October 1968. By then, J-M was the largest asbestos company in the United States, nearing one billion dollars in sales. The complaint, in part, stated: "In the operation of its aforesaid plant in Manville, New Jersey, did knowingly, or with reason to know, caused asbestos dust and fumes to be admitted into the atmosphere and become airborne, constituting a continual invasion of the surrounding area and locality, including the resident areas of the community. . . . The Defendant knew and had reason to know of the high degree of risk of health others and the residents in the surrounding area of the plant . . . and therefore became strictly liable for the decedent's ultimate injury and death."

What followed in the memo was an astounding condemnation

of the company for whom the town had been named. "In the Fetchko case, it is felt we have no chance of winning when it is litigated since it is evident that Johns-Manville had contaminated both air and water in the past. In fact a Johns-Manville attorney stated, 'Confidentially, Johns-Manville has been contaminating the "Hell" out of both the air and the water for quite some time.' It is apparent Johns-Manville is concerned and frightened over the implications."

As many insurers had predicted, the ten- to forty-year latency period that, in part, allowed the asbestos companies to expose its workers and consumers to fibers and get away with it for as long as they did was coming back to haunt them. Even as J-M and other asbestos companies began to claim they had discontinued use of asbestos, they faced the beginning of a tide of plaintiff claims that was just starting to grow because their victims would be getting sick for the next forty years.

In 1977, the asbestos industry and their insurers made the critical decision not to admit liability. It was a gamble because the few legal cases that had already been tried had resulted in verdicts going to both sides. It wasn't until a few years later, when the number of lawsuits grew from a few hundred to tens and then hundreds of thousands, that the industry realized it had made a serious mistake.

The workers hardest hit during the four decades from 1940 to 1980 were shipyard laborers, who began falling victim to asbestos-related diseases by the hundreds of thousands. This time the cover-up wasn't orchestrated as much by the asbestos industry as by the U.S. Navy. In fact, the navy's role in the asbestos cover-up may be the darkest hour of its entire history. To date, the navy has neither admitted its role nor taken any steps to ameliorate the immense damage for which it was directly responsible during those years.

The use of asbestos on military vessels skyrocketed during the frantic effort to restore America's fleet, which had been damaged at Pearl Harbor. The total employment in the U.S. shipyards jumped from about 170,000 workers before WWII to nearly 2 million by 1944. At least 4.5 million shipyard workers were exposed during that time, according to then-Secretary of Health, Education and Welfare Joe Califano Jr., and millions more were exposed after the war until asbestos use in shipyards declined in the late 1970s.

Experienced seafarers say that the most fearful event onboard ship isn't sinking but fire. Beginning in the 1930s, the maritime industry sought to make ships fireproof by packing everything possible, including pipes, engines, turbines, boilers, and heaters, with asbestos. This required a vast amount of asbestos insulation because most ships and submarines contained miles cf piping. For nearly fifty years, asbestos blankets and molds were used on virtually every ship. In addition, asbestos sprays were liberally applied to most ships to fireproof the inside of the bulkheads, decks, and cabins.

The enclosed quarters inside the ships were the worst possible environment for asbestos workers. Many of the men and women who worked belowdecks were subjected to huge quantities of fibers in a short time. To make matters worse, amosite and crocidolite, which are particularly deadly forms of asbestos, were frequently used.

By the onset of WWII, so much had been written about the adverse health effects of asbestos that the navy was forced to take notice of the potential dangers. In December 1942, Phillip Drinker of the Harvard School of Public Health made a presentation before the U.S. Maritime Commission on the minimum requirements for safety in shipyards. A large number of insurance company representatives attended due to increasing concerns over the potential liability of the asbestos industry.

"Asbestosis is caused in connection with the handling of as-bestos," Drinker told the audience. "This is not unlike silicosis in its effects, and we rather expect it to occur in shipyards, because we have seen asbestos being handled in installation work with little or no precautions."

Despite the warnings, the navy and the shipyard operators failed to fully protect the workers. The history of these failures was chronicled, in part, in a series of articles written by Bill Burke, an in-vestigative reporter for the Hampton Roads, Virginia–based news-paper, *The Virginia-Pilot*, in 2001. After reviewing the navy's actions during the early 1940s, Burke wrote: "In 1943, the government is-sued standards intended to protect a shipyard force that labored 24 hours a day, seven days a week in massive fogs of asbestos dust. But, more than three decades would pass before the government would begin enforcing those standards and take steps to protect workers."

Former shipyard worker David Durham told Burke that as a teenager he worked during the war helping to fit thermal asbestos insulation onto the networks of pipes that carried cold water and steam throughout the ship. Durham also tore off old insulation so machinists and boilermakers could make repairs. They worked in hot engine rooms and boiler rooms that were dense with asbestos dust. At the end of the day, the men were covered with it. "You'd just knock it off your ears," Durham said.

Durham remembered one old worker who assured him that the asbestos dust was harmless. Much of the asbestos went into making a light cement material called boiler composition that con-sisted of 85 percent magnesium and 15 percent asbestos. Clearly, the old worker had been told about only part of the ingredients. He told Durham the concoction was just the same as milk of magnesia, with just a little asbestos in it. He then popped some in his mouth and swallowed it.

The insulation, cloth, and bags of dry asbestos-containing cement the workers handled contained no warning labels, even though they were made to the navy's exact specifications.

While only about one out of every five hundred workers in the shipyards was an "asbestos worker," most of the people who helped build the ships—welders, carpenters, painters, sheet metal workers, riggers, pipe fitters, electricians, and other construction workers— were exposed to asbestos at one time or another. What they didn't know was that working in American shipyards during WWII proved to be as deadly as fighting in the war. During WWII, 16.1 million Americans were in the Armed Services, according to the U.S. Department of Defense. The combat death rate was about eighteen soldiers per thousand. The asbestos-related death rate among wartime shipyard employees was about fourteen per thousand. Because of the traditional underreporting of asbestosis deaths, the death rate is likely much higher.

It is perhaps one of humanity's darkest comedies to think that countries can spend billions of dollars developing the most highly sophisticated weapons of death on the planet and yet, in the end, the tiny asbestos fiber turned out to be a more efficient killer.

American veterans' groups around the country are angry and frustrated that the U.S. Navy has never admitted to any culpability involving asbestos exposures. It was as if the navy looked at shipyard workers as they did combat soldiers—some were expected to sacrifice for their country. The only difference was that soldiers knew the dangers that awaited them—and they were looked upon as heroes by their country. Shipyard workers were never told about their "enemy," and they have been ignored by the government and the country they served.

The orders to ignore the dangers of asbestos came from the top levels. Barry Castleman uncovered a memo from C. S. Stephenson,

U.S. Navy Commander of Preventive Medicine, to Rear Admiral Ross McIntire, on March 11, 1941, that showed the decision came from the Oval Office.

Under the head "Asbestosis," the memo stated: "We are not protecting the men as we should." It then referred to the objections by the navy to having teams of Public Health Service scientists studying the working conditions of the shipyard employees. "I told [the assistant secretary of the navy] that I had spoken to you and that you had indicated that President Roosevelt thought that it might not be the best policy, due to the fact that they might cause disturbances in the labor element."

The navy also chose to continue to ignore warnings from some of the most renowned physicians of the time that the working conditions in the shipyards would lead to significant numbers of asbestosis and cancer cases. As a result, the exposures continued long after WWII. Korea and Vietnam–era shipbuilders and sailors were continually exposed to asbestos-laden ships. Tom Van Noord, now a Placerville, California, attorney, served in the Merchant Marines during the Vietnam War. He worked with asbestos nearly every day as his ship brought supplies to the troops in Saigon.

"Whenever we had to fix the pipes or the machinery, we just tore the asbestos away and stuffed it in fifty-five-gallon drums with our hands," he said. "Nobody said anything to us about it being dangerous." Van Noord said he knows the odds are he will ultimately suffer from an asbestos-related disease. "I try not to think about it, but it's just a waiting game now," he said.

Charles Ay of Orange County, California, is an expert on how careless the U.S. Navy can be. Ay lost his father, two uncles, and a brother-in-law to asbestos-related diseases, and a second brother-in-law has been diagnosed with asbestosis. They all worked at the

Long Beach, California, shipyards, building ships primarily for the navy. Ay, who worked as an insulator in federal shipyards from 1960 through 1981, also has the disease.

"Oh, the navy did its job carefully; they simply sent out specifications to the shipbuilders and were careful not to use the word 'asbestos,'" he said. "Did the navy know? Yes. Should they have stopped the use of it? Absolutely. Everybody is dirty in this business."

Ay, an outspoken opponent of asbestos use, worked from 1971 to 1981 as the business manager of the Asbestos Workers Union Local 20. "The problem we had in those days was in understanding the disease," he said. "We all heard that cigarettes were bad for you, but the asbestos industry advertised heavily that asbestos wasn't a problem. When information did start leaking out that asbestos was dangerous, the companies used words like 'pneumoconiosis' to describe the adverse health effects. That may as well have been Russian to us. They also told us to wear respirators, but it was a rule they never enforced."

Ay believes there was only one reason the navy and its contractors allowed workers to be so readily exposed to the fibers. "Money. It's pretty simple, really." Ay, who has testified in asbestos legal suits about conditions in the shipyards, said that by 1975 so much was known about asbestos hazards that to fully protect a worker the companies would have had to purchase HazMat suits, much like the EPA inspectors now wear in suspected asbestos-polluted areas.

"By the time you add up the cost of all that protective gear, you are talking about hundreds of thousands of dollars a day to protect all the people that work in shipyards," Ay said. "It was a lot cheaper to let them work unprotected. The companies figured, 'Sure, some of the workers will die and fewer will sue us—it is still much cheaper than buying the protective gear.'"

Ay, who now operates a marine asbestos inspection business,

said it is difficult sometimes to think of his father and the other family members he has lost. "I struggled for a period to get a handle on my anger," he said. "Rage does nothing. People won't listen to you, and you can become a bitter, isolated person."

Asked if he had vanquished all his anger, Ay paused for a long moment. "No," he said. "It will never all be gone. The part that does make me mad is that someone took away our right to make a reasonable decision about our own lives. If they had just told us about the dangers up front, we could have made our own decisions about whether we wanted to work there. But I guess that's what they were afraid we would do."

7

DEATH BY MILLIONS OF CUTS

The effects of asbestos fibers on the human body are varied and complex. Doctors now know that they are the primary if not sole cause of mesothelioma, the terrible, fatal cancer that races out of the lining of the stomach or lungs and can attack the ribs, diaphragm, spine, and heart. According to physicians at the Mesothelioma Applied Research Foundation (MARF), an organization of some of the most respected doctors and scientists in the nation, "Although there is no universal standard for measuring 'suffering,' we submit that on a scale of 0 to 100, mesothelioma patients—who experience severe suffering not only of a physical nature but also from emotional trauma due to inadequate and uncertain therapies—typically are at the highest range of this scale."

Dr. Alan Whitehouse, a Spokane, Washington, physician who called asbestos diseases "much worse than AIDS," believes that with proper funding for research, treatments can be developed. Yet as of today, there is no treatment and precious little knowledge about why asbestos fibers affect humans the way they do. A few scientists and physicians, usually working with meager budgets, are attempting to follow the clues deep into molecular levels. Despite these medical efforts, perhaps the most succinct appraisal of the effect of the microscopic spearlike fibers was offered by Bob Wilkins, who has advanced asbestosis. "First, they leave you short of breath, like a bear squeezing you; then they begin to cause you constant pain; then they usually kill you."

The microscopic fibers—if you can see one it is too big to hurt you—also cause asbestosis and lung cancer. Studies show it is also a cause of cancer of the stomach, colon-rectum, larynx, pharynx, kidneys, and esophagus. Moreover, autopsies have located asbestos fibers in the brain, bone marrow, large and small intestines, spleen, pancreas, prostate, thyroid, bladder, and liver. They can also be passed from mother to fetus.

"In Asia they had a medieval torture called Death by a Thousand Cuts," said the U.S. Public Health Service's Aubrey Miller. "This is death by millions of cuts. Once inside the lungs, each little fiber causes tiny scars as your body sends out cells to attack the fibers. Human lungs are tough, they can handle a lot of things, and most of the time can take care of foreign particles. But asbestos fibers don't dissolve, and they are not easily removed. They are among the most durable substances in the world; that's why asbestos has been used in so many products. Asbestos fibers can stay in your lungs for decades after exposure and cause disease and death."

Physicians and scientists predict that nearly 40 percent of workers and others who have multiple exposures to asbestos fibers will die from asbestos-caused cancer. Another significant percentage of those exposed will die of asbestosis. Although these staggering numbers have been known for some time by corporate and government experts, one of the reasons asbestos remains a ubiquitous element in products today is that few people outside a handful of doctors, scientists, and victims are aware of the massive damage it can cause in the human body.

Conferences like the New Directions and Needs in Asbestos

Research Conference held in Missoula, Montana, in the summer of 2002 help physicians share information, but far more must be done in terms of research before the epidemiology of the asbestos diseases are fully understood. The sad fact is that asbestos victims have been so completely neglected to such a degree that there is no cure for any of the myriad asbestos-caused diseases. These are devastating illnesses that cause the human body to waste away, the victims suffering not only from the physical pain but also the knowledge that more money is spent trying to prevent cat leukemia or in the construction of one stealth bomber than on finding a cure.

"We aren't looking for the number of mesothelioma and other asbestos-related diseases to level off until the year 2047," Henry Falk, the assistant administrator of the Agency for Toxic Substances and Disease Registry (ATSDR), told the Missoula conferees. "We need to find a treatment for these diseases, or we are going to have a tremendous number of sick and dying people on our hands."

No scientific discussion about the ravages of the fibers, regardless of the dire number of victims projected in the near future, has the emotional impact of visiting Libby. Contrary to some colorful media accounts, people are not dropping dead on street corners; nor do you see a large number of portable oxygen tanks, although they are present around the town. It is when you sit and talk with some of those who are suffering that you realize the extent to which asbestos has affected their lives.

Helen Bundrock lives just down the street from Wilkins. The two are neighbors, sharing the same apartment complex. They also share something else—advanced cases of asbestosis caused by the tremolite contamination from the W. R. Grace mine.

Bundrock, an attractive woman with middle-aged children, is astonishingly cheerful. Happiness seems to be her true nature, and even the events in Libby have not managed to take that away from her. She talked glowingly and with love about her five children. Then she mentioned that all of them have been diagnosed with asbestos diseases.

"My oldest daughter is fifty-three, and she has asbestosis," Bundrock said. "She has good days and bad days. My son has it; he worked at the mine for twenty years. We thought our youngest daughter had escaped it, but when she came home from Phoenix where she lives now there was a letter waiting for her. She had been screened here, and they asked her to come back for a CAT scan. That's when we knew." The entire family was poisoned by the asbestos dust that Helen's husband, Art, brought home during the years he worked at the vermiculite mine.

Helen paused for a breath with almost every word as she described how she used to wash Art's dirty work clothes in an old ringer washing machine that got so clogged with asbestos dust that she had to clean out the drain with each washing.

"Art was a fun person to be around," she said. "We had so much fun together. He was one of the first of the mine workers to be diagnosed. I remember the doctor at the time asking Art if he had any grandchildren. At the time we only had one granddaughter, and the doctor said: 'I'm going to get you away from that mine so you can enjoy her.' He wouldn't even let Art go back to the mine to get his tools because there was still so much asbestos up there."

Although the conversation was clearly a labor for Bundrock, she was determined to tell the story and refused to reach for the oxygen bottle that sat nearby. By the end of the story she coughed nearly nonstop. It wasn't the hacking, violent cough of cigarette smokers, but a shallow, shuddering convulsion done with eyes shut tight in an attempt to deal with the pain.

Helen's children can watch her disease progress to see what is in store for them. So can her twenty-two-year-old grandson, who used to play in the vermiculite piles near the Libby ball fields. He was diagnosed with asbestos disease last year.

"I will say one thing about the people at W. R. Grace," Bundrock said. "I can't help but feel sorry for them. I know when this life is over that we answer to somebody. I feel better in my shoes than in theirs. They have a lot to answer for."

Science does not know yet why some asbestos exposures lead to the advent of mesothelioma. It may have to do with the size and type of fibers that invade the membrane linings of the lung and stomach. Other factors may include the number of fibers inhaled or the DNA makeup and age of the victim. People exposed when they are young seem especially susceptible to mesothelioma and other asbestos diseases. One thing is certain: Mesothelioma is deadly, usually killing its victim in from two months to three years from the time most symptoms appear. Cigarette smoking does not seem to be a factor in its development.

News reporters, governmental brochures, and even some scientists continue to call mesothelioma a rare form of cancer. Unfortunately, while that may have been true years ago, today there are thousands of new cases per year in the industrialized world. In the United States alone, up to nine thousand new cases a year are expected, according to medical experts. The number is similar in western Europe, where more than a quarter of a million victims may die from the disease in the next thirty-five years, according to Professor Julian Peto of the Institute of Cancer Research and the London School of Hygiene and Tropical Medicine. "The figures are horrifying," Peto told the BBC. "The cancer was extremely rare and now it has become common, and will become more common."

Australia, too, is expecting an epidemic of mesothelioma cases. More Australians now die of mesothelioma than of cervical cancer.

The only known cause of mesothelioma is exposure to asbestos fibers. Some scientists, especially those employed by the asbestos industry, have attempted to point to other causal factors, but most experts believe asbestos is the singular cause.

"All mesotheliomas are caused by asbestos," said Dr. Whitehouse flatly. "If someone has the disease and you haven't found any exposure to asbestos, you haven't looked hard enough. It is a horrible disease with a terrible death. It is the most miserable cancer I deal with."

Mesothelioma, which is noncontagious, usually occurs in two places within the human body. The most common type is pleural mesothelioma, which is a cancer of the cells that make up the pleura or lining around the outside of the lungs and inside of the ribs. It accounts for about 75 percent of all cases.

Pleural mesothelioma is not a symptomatic disease until late in its course. It often takes from twenty to forty years for symptoms to appear. In 1988, the mean patient age for mesothelioma patients was in the low- to mid-seventies, but that has come down steadily to the mid-fifties. Even people in their twenties and thirties are now coming down with the disease, having been exposed as infants or small children. The symptoms include shortness of breath, weakness, appetite and weight loss, chest pains, lower back pains, persistent coughing, and difficulty in swallowing. There is often a buildup of a bloody fluid in the pleural lining between the lungs and chest wall.

What pleural mesothelioma usually hides for years is a buildup of a slender, sheeted tumor that often grows to the size of a thin pillow. When it is finally detected by an X ray or CAT scan, it is not unusual for the physician and the victim to be stunned by the size of the tumor, which doesn't present itself well because it does not grow in the telltale lumps of other cancers. The actual diagnosis of mesothelioma is usually done through a biopsy. Most physicians are not yet familiar with it and frequently misdiagnose it, even after death.

The spread of the tumor also usually causes scarring, or pleural thickening. This reduces the flexibility of the elastic membrane and restricts the victim's ability to breathe properly. The tumor can spread in any direction. It can wrap around a victim's heart, or it can grow inward and slowly crush the lungs. It becomes especially painful when it expands outward to the chest wall and ribs.

Asbestos also causes peritoneal mesothelioma, a cancer of the mesothelial cells in the peritoneal membrane of the abdomen. Like pleural mesothelioma, this cancer is slow growing most of the time but is usually well advanced and moving quickly by the time symptoms are noticed. These include stomach pains, weakness, weight and appetite loss, nausea, and swelling. The tumor is invasive, often blocking and distending the bowel. If the tumor grows upward, it can hinder breathing. As it grows, it can cause intense pain.

Most of the treatments involve pain reduction, although a process called "debulking" is used occasionally to remove large pieces of the tumor to relieve pressure on the body's primary organs and the chest wall. Rib resection, muscle cutting and spreading, and placement of tubes in cavities are sometimes done to relieve interior pressure, but those are highly invasive maneuvers that usually leave the patient in discomfort for some time after the operation. Radiation and chemotherapy are also used to reduce the tumor.

If all this sounds gruesome, it is. But these are the types of choices and procedures that tens of thousands of victims now face and that generations of victims, some not yet born, will continue to face if people continue to be exposed to asbestos.

Since asbestos fibers are generally inhaled, they must take a circuitous route to get to the abdomen. Scientists believe that some of the fibers may be caught by the mucus of the trachea and bronchi and end up being swallowed. A second route may be that fibers lodged in the lungs can move into the lymphatic system and be transported to the peritoneum. However they get there, they spear cells and can damage DNA as well as release the cell's destructive cellular enzymes that in turn damage other cells.

Asbestosis, a scarring process caused in the interstitial, or inner part of the lung, by the body's attempt to attack the fibers, is the most common disease caused by asbestos exposure. It is progressive and can develop fully in as little as seven years and cause death in as little as thirteen years. In other cases, it can take twenty years or more before its victims begin to feel symptoms. The disease process begins after the fibers are inhaled and escape the body's natural defense system because of their thin, tiny size. They travel into the lungs and often pierce one of the three hundred million gas-exchanging structures called alveoli deep within the lungs. Much of the current molecular research being done on asbestos surrounds disease-fighting cells within each alveolus, called macrophages.

Macrophages attack the fibers much like the body attacks a splinter in a finger. Unfortunately, they are no match for the mineral asbestos fibers, which are too long and too tough for the body to dissolve or absorb. The macrophages generally tear themselves open trying to "eat" the fibers, and their destructive, digestive molecules spill out, causing more tissue damage. The body quickly heals the microscopic injuries, but scar tissue, called fibrosis, develops. In the end, it is the cumulative buildup of this pulmonary fibrosis that can ultimately disable and kill its host. At the same time, the fibers become coated with layers of protein and iron. These tiny lumps are called asbestos bodies.

The fibrosis causes the lining of the air sacs to thicken and stiffen, making it difficult for the body to pass oxygen to the bloodstream and to properly rid itself (through exhaling) of the buildup of carbon dioxide. As the scarring process, which is progressive and irreversible, continues, the victim begins to slowly suffocate. The coughing impulse that usually can rid the lungs of unwanted debris is triggered almost continuously, but the fibers have penetrated too deeply and cannot be dislodged.

Asbestosis attacks both lungs. It is usually concentrated in the lower part of the lungs, but it ultimately invades the entire lung. It is not a cancer and it is not contagious, and many victims live with it for years, although at any time it can suddenly speed up and cause death.

The disease is usually diagnosed through the evaluation of the victim's exposure history, the scarring and thickening that can be seen on X rays and CAT scans, and the victim's reduced ability on a pulmonary function test. Typical symptoms include shortness of breath, a persistent dry cough, sometimes pain in the upper chest and back, weight loss, and occasionally a "clubbing" of fingers and toes that results from lack of oxygen. Physicians familiar with the disease often say that when they use a stethoscope on the lower lungs of asbestosis victims, their breathing sounds like Velcro opening.

"It can be extremely painful," said Pat Cohen, clinic coordinator for Libby's Center for Asbestos-Related Diseases (CARD). "Every time a patient with asbestosis takes a breath—which happens about sixteen to twenty times a minute—it rubs a sore spot. Your lungs just can't expand. You may be okay watching television, but if you get up to get yourself a cup of coffee in the kitchen, you suddenly run out of breath. Many asbestosis victims can't even get across the room. They sleep in a chair at night so they can breathe. It is a slow, strangulating process, and there is nothing anybody can do about it."

Because asbestosis can severely limit the amount of oxygen sent to the rest of the body, it can have a devastating effect on organs such as the heart. Many people with asbestosis develop cor pulmonale—right-sided heart failure—which is often deadly. Most physicians now believe that asbestos-caused deaths are significantly underreported because many asbestosis victims actually die of heart attacks and other causes. Unless physicians are aware of the insidious and chameleonlike nature of the symptoms of asbestosis (and relatively few are), the real culprit—asbestos fibers—is frequently overlooked as the official cause of death.

For reasons that are yet unclear to physicians, the combination of smoking and inhalation of asbestos exponentially increases a person's chance of dying of lung cancer. It is one of the most lethal combination of factors known on earth. Scientists believe that smokers who are exposed to asbestos at relatively high levels run an eight to ten times greater risk of developing lung cancer than smokers in the general population with little or no asbestos exposure. The combination of asbestos and tobacco is like "throwing gasoline on oily rags and putting a match to them," according to one scientist. Just why the two substances act like a bomb within the human body is not yet known.

The official cause of death among those who died of lung cancer—even though they smoked and had high asbestos exposures—is nearly always attributed to smoking alone. It is yet another reason asbestos-related deaths are underreported.

Most physicians believe that it may take less exposure to asbestos fibers to cause cancer than to cause asbestosis. Besides lung cancer and mesothelioma, asbestos spears can cause cell and DNA mutations in several of the major bodily organs. Up to 10 percent of asbestos workers die of gastrointestinal cancer, which is a general term for several different cancers of the digestive system. It includes cancers of the esophagus, stomach, colon, and rectum. These cancers, nearly all of them deadly, are thought to be associated with swallowing the asbestos fibers, which is a reason to review the current assumption that drinking asbestos-contaminated water is harmless.

Scientists are not certain, but some believe the fibers may migrate out of the pleural linings of the lungs into these other areas. Research has shown that asbestos fibers carried throughout the lymphatic system can also cause cancer in the kidneys. Although rare, asbestos fibers can also cause tonsil and tongue cancer and testicular cancer.

One of the most controversial medical aspects of asbestos poisoning has to do with something called pleural disease. This is caused by fibrosis within the thin pleural lining of the lung. The lining has a slick, lubricated surface that allows normal lungs to easily expand and contract. As the inhaled fibers move from the lung to the pleura—pulled there by the constant expansion and contraction of the lung—the scarring they leave behind causes the pleura to thicken, robbing the lungs of their elasticity. This causes intense pain in many patients and can ultimately cause death. Pleural plaques, which are hardened fibrous little plates of tissues that form on the pleural surface, also result from the fibers. They are similar in texture to cartilage and are considered telltale markers by physicians that the patient has been exposed to asbestos.

The controversy comes from industry and media sources and even some plaintiff lawyers who argue that pleural disease is benign. They believe that victims, whose only symptom of asbestos exposure are these markers, are not truly sick and should therefore not be allowed to sue over their exposure. The asbestos industry has long claimed that a majority of cases involve people with "only" pleural disease. Their arguments have been trumpeted by a number of national media outlets—some of which are owned by large corporations that are themselves being sued over asbestos exposures—and by some plaintiff law firms that represent only people with advanced asbestos-related diseases such as mesothelioma. The mesothelioma cases are traditionally awarded one million dollars or more by juries. With more than fifty corporations already filing for protection from the onslaught of asbestos lawsuits under Chapter 11, these plaintiff attorneys fear the funds for the "truly sick" victims of asbestos exposure may soon run out.

On the other side of the argument are physicians who believe strongly that pleural disease is a serious threat to human life. For example, Dr. Whitehouse, who has treated nearly 450 asbestos victims from Libby, told the audience at the 2002 Missoula asbestos conference, "Pleural disease is progressive. It is not benign, whether pleural plaque or pleural thickening." He said the events in Libby must serve as a "wake-up call" regarding the seriousness of pleural disease. "We demonstrated in a hundred and twenty cases in Libby that pleural disease victims are losing their pulmonary function at three percent per year," Dr. Whitehouse said. "We can no longer say, 'This is just pleural thickening or pleural plaquing.' People who are minimizing this disease are putting their heads in the sand."

Another of the multitude of elements of asbestos we still do not understand is the level of exposure that is dangerous for humans. Much of the older, traditional literature, including brochures from governmental sources—even one from the ATSDR—still insists that exposure becomes "a health concern when asbestos fibers are breathed in at high concentrations over a long period of time." Certainly, autopsies have shown that asbestos victims often have hundreds of millions of fibers in their lungs. Research and the events in Libby, however, have indicated that this adage, while true in the majority of cases, has many exceptions. Studies have proven that animals have developed mesothelioma after only one day of exposure, and asbestos-related diseases have appeared in people in Libby, and in many other areas, who have had only brief, if high-intensity, exposures to asbestos.

Because asbestos fibers do not often break down inside the body, they have a cumulative effect over the life of the patient. Although one fiber can damage the DNA of any given cell, it is generally thought that the more fibers inside a patient's lung, the more chance there is for an advanced disease over time. It is also likely, however, that the type and size of the fibers also play a critical role in the pathology. Moreover, it is difficult many times to determine how many fibers a worker or consumer may be exposed to at any one given time. Billions of fibers can exist in a work site or home area, but if they are not disturbed, the chance of a sizable exposure is small, even over extended periods of time. That is not a practical scenario, however, since fibers are easily released from friable asbestos materials and even the slightest of movements can send millions of the lightweight fibers into the air. Even one exposure in a contaminated area can cause a massive inhalation of fibers, especially in enclosed spaces such as attics.

Events in Libby have helped break down the lasting myth that one must encounter "lengthy, high-dose exposures" to fall victim to the fibers. For example, one victim of asbestos from Libby, an accountant, recently died of an asbestos-related disease even though his only known exposure was during the two months he spent working at a vermiculite expanding plant when he was seventeen years old. Another Libby victim had no known exposure pathways except for the fact that she worked in a local chiropractor's office and often hung up the dusty coats of the men who came straight from work at the vermiculite mine. Her exposure time was brief, but the number of fibers she was subjected to was most likely extremely high.

Perhaps the most bitter dispute between scientists—which left doctors and researchers slinging accusations at each other throughout the 1980s and 1990s—has been over the relative dangers of the different "types" of asbestos. Officially, *asbestos* is the term given to a group of six fibrous, crystalline minerals commonly used commercially. The debate begins with this definition because there are several hundred types of similar fibrous minerals that many scientists believe are equally as dangerous to human health. Because the federal government has not included these in the definition of asbestos, however, these minerals, many of which can be found in marble and talc, for example, are not recognized as "dangerous" by the U.S. government and are therefore not regulated.

The six types of recognized asbestos are chrysotile, crocidolite, amosite, anthophyllite, actinolite, and tremolite. All of these occur naturally in the environment, but that doesn't mean they are benign. Poisonous snakes and noxious gases occur naturally, too, but they certainly are not safe to be around.

Chrysotile, which is predominately white in color, accounts for the vast majority of the asbestos used commercially. Crocidolite, or blue asbestos, and amosite, which has brown fibers, were used extensively on ships and for spray-on insulation products. Anthophyllite, a gray asbestos, is also used commercially. Actinolite and tremolite are considered contaminates and have never been used commercially to any degree.

The real debate over these asbestos types came from the differences in the fibers between chrysotile and the others. Chrysotile, which is still heavily mined in Canada, Russia, China, and many other countries, comes from a serpentine rock which describes the shape of its fibers—curled like a serpent. The only operating asbestos mine in the United States (which is in California, where serpentine is the state rock) is a chrysotile mine.

The other asbestos types—called amphiboles—have more rigid fibers. Tremolite, actinolite, and anthophyllite are common rocks that occur in solid or "nonasbestiform" structures that do not shed fibers, as well as in the deadly asbestiform structures. For decades, scientists and physicians have debated over the relative dangers of chrysotile asbestos. The industry still calls chrysotile the "environmentally friendly mineral." It has become clear, however, that the industry, faced with growing proof that its product causes asbestos-related diseases, sought to use the deadly nature of the amphibole fibers as a "promotable villain" to deflect criticism from the harmful effects of the chrysotile fibers. Since WWII, some industry sources—despite an avalanche of studies to the contrary—continually provided the public message that chrysotile was the "good asbestos" and had fibers that could be absorbed successfully by the human body. The industry blamed the tremendous number of deaths in the Canadian chrysotile mines and elsewhere on tremolite and other amphibole contamination of the chrysotile.

Amphiboles made good villains because products containing them make up a relatively small portion of the market and are usually sold in Third World countries that offer the least resistance in terms of environmental and worker safety and product laws. Given the fact that thousands of products containing chrysotile are still legal in the United States, and given the asbestos industry's determination to further penetrate Third World markets and in some cases move their manufacturing centers to these regions, the debate over chrysotile remains literally a life-or-death issue for perhaps millions of people.

In the eyes of most worldwide experts, there should be no such debate. Nearly all credible private researchers, as well as most governmental and public health agencies, have concluded that chrysotile is a highly dangerous substance. Leading the condemnation of chrysotile has been the Mount Sinai Medical Center researchers and doctors. In a report prepared for the New York Academy of Sciences, John Harington of the Department of Community and Preventive Medicine at Mount Sinai, wrote:

> *Chrysotile has developed an unwarranted reputation for being the least troublesome of the fibrous asbestos minerals, the amphiboles having largely attracted the most attention. . . . [However,] there is consistent evidence that chrysotile is as active as crocidolite and amosite in inducing both lung cancer and mesothelioma. It is also substantially clear from the best available evidence of studies of human experience associated with exposure to chrysotile that this form of asbestos is carcinogenic to humans.*

In a 1999 article in *Industrial Health Magazine*, Dr. Philip Landrigan, Dr. William Nicholson, and Dr. Yasunosuke Suzuki from Mount Sinai, and Dr. Joseph Ladou of the University of California at San Francisco, stated that:

> *Clinical and epidemiologic studies have established incontrovertibly that chrysotile causes cancer of the lung, malignant mesothelioma of the pleura and peritoneum, cancer of the larynx and certain gastrointestinal cancers. Chrysotile*

*also causes asbestosis. . . . Comparative analyses have es-
tablished that chrysotile is 2 to 4 times less potent than crocidolite asbestos in its ability to cause malignant
mesothelioma, but of equal potency of causation of lung
cancer. . . . Chrysotile asbestos is an important cause of
human illness and death.*

Numerous other studies and agencies debunk the so-called
chrysotile defense.

- "The claim that various types of asbestos differ in their
  hazard is particularly insidious. It is put forth by the manufacturers of Canadian asbestos [chrysotile], the type of asbestos most widely used in New York, and throughout the
  United States. The central claim is [that chrysotile] is harmless. However, that claim is not based on fact, and it is not
  supported by the results of epidemiological and toxicolog-
  ical studies conducted in the U.S. and overseas. These
  studies show that all types of asbestos . . . are fully capable
  of producing the full spectrum of asbestos-related diseases."
  *(Bold, Bianci DeVito, Landrigan, Pettengil, Second Annual Re-
  port, State of New York Asbestos Advisory Board, February
  1990.)*
- OSHA, the EPA, the U.S. Department of Health and Human
  Services, and NIOSH (the National Institute for Occupational
  Safety and Health) all have stated that chrysotile asbestos is a
  great hazard to human health and causes a variety of
  asbestos-related diseases.
- In 1998, the Canadian asbestos industry, stung when France,
  one of its primary customers, banned asbestos altogether, appealed to the World Trade Organization to strike the ban.
  Their argument centered on the relative "safety" of chrysotile

asbestos. The WTO formed an international panel to investigate. In 2000, the panel's final report was crushing to Canadian hopes. The panel report stated: "The carcinogenicity of chrysotile fibres has been acknowledged for some time by international bodies. This carcinogenicity was confirmed by the experts consulted by the Panel, with respect to both lung cancers and mesotheliomas, even though the experts appear to acknowledge that chrysotile is less likely to cause mesotheliomas than amphiboles. We also note that the experts confirmed that the types of cancer concerned had a mortality rate of close to 100 percent. We therefore consider that we have sufficient evidence that there is in fact a serious carcinogenic risk associated with the inhalation of chrysotile fibres." *(World Trade Organization, European Communities—Measures Affecting Asbestos and Asbestos-Containing Products, Report of the Panel, paragraph 8.188, September 18, 2000.)*

- "I note that there has been some discussion that chrysotile wasn't nearly as dangerous as some of the other fibers. Tell that to our widows. Approximately 90 percent of the asbestosis incurred by our membership has been through exposure to chrysotile. If there is something more dangerous than chrysotile, we don't want to meet it." *(Edward J. Carlough, of the Sheet Metal Worker's International Association, speaking at the 1991 Third Wave of Asbestos Disease conference sponsored by the New York Academy of Sciences.)*

- "With regard to an increased risk of lung cancer in chrysotile workers, experience of Quebec chrysotile miners and chrysotile textile workers has clearly indicated that there are increased risks with increasing levels of exposure." *(Dr. Graham Gibbs, on behalf of the government of Alberta, Canada, speaking at the 1991 Third Wave of Asbestos Disease conference sponsored by the New York Academy of Sciences.)*

• Separate studies in Italy, Germany, Zimbabwe, China, Quebec, and several in the United States have all concluded that chrysotile causes the entire spectrum of asbestos-related diseases, including mesothelioma.

To underscore a point already made in this book: Today, despite the terrible human cost of asbestos-related diseases, there are no cures, and very little research money is being spent to find them.

"Asbestos causes some of the worst cancers, and there isn't much you can do for patients," said Dr. Robert Cameron, head of thoracic oncology at the UCLA Medical Center. "Right now our treatments are almost as bad as the disease. In Europe, they just tell people with mesothelioma to go home; there isn't anything that can be done for them. At least in the U.S. we have people who are trying to develop therapies."

Dr. Cameron said he knows of a private pharmaceutical company that had some initial success curing mesothelioma in mice. "The problem is the drug was purchased by a company in San Diego, California, that is interested in using it in another area," he said. "Most drug companies, like most people, have never heard of mesothelioma so they don't look at mesothelioma patients as a customer source."

"A great starting point would be for doctors throughout the country to begin to understand what a widespread problem asbestos-related disease is," said Libby's Pat Cohen. "Very few doctors even recognize the symptoms. If we caught the diseases earlier, there may be something we could do."

Cohen, who has seen hundreds of cases in Libby, where many of the patients have become her friends, said there is a distinct pat-

tern of physical decline among those with asbestosis. "The first step
in the process is usually ibuprofen," she said. "If they turn their head
or breathe wrong it can really cause pain. After that come ice packs
and hot packs and then more serious and powerful painkillers. At
that point, even getting a cold or the flu can be life-threatening.
Their lungs can fill up with fluid and have to be drained. As their
ability to breathe becomes increasingly impaired, they end up being
forced to use oxygen. Death usually comes when the brain, heart, or
whichever organ gives out first, fails."

Cohen has watched dozens of her friends put up courageous
battles against the disease. "You can't believe how brave these people
are," she said. "I know what real courage is. I've seen it many times
in Libby, Montana."

Although he looks lean and strong, Les Skramstad's lungs are
severely compromised, and he has difficulty walking from the
restaurant to the car. He has to rest against the newspaper stand, and
he tilts his cap back, quietly gasping for breath. Somehow he man-
ages to do it all with dignity and grace. "I won't do the oxygen," he
says. "Once you do the oxygen, you're in trouble. I'm not going to
do it. I'm going to fight it as long as I can."

Perhaps the most poignant picture of how asbestosis ravages a
human life can be seen in a remarkable documentary feature on
Libby and the Grace mine, called *Dust to Dust*, produced by Michael
Brown of Dallas. The entire film is a gripping chronicle of the poisoning of the town, but especially moving is a piece of home video
shot by Gayla Benefield of her mother, Margaret. Once an upbeat,
energetic woman, Margaret's tiny figure is curled up in bed as she
suffers from the latter stages of the disease. The blanket is pulled to
her chin. She looks small enough to lift with one hand. She talks

with great difficulty. Her eyes are shut with pain behind glasses that look oversized on her face.

"You just couldn't get enough breath," she says in a voice barely audible. "You coughed all the time." Gayla's voice then intercedes as Margaret begins to cough. The noise is small and desperate, like a child's. Gayla explains that her mother has spent the last year and a half in bed. Before the widespread asbestos problems in Libby were known, a Libby doctor originally diagnosed Margaret with lung cancer. He opened Margaret's lungs and found not lung cancer but two sections of plaque the size of saucers.

As Gayla talks, her mother moans softly, raises her knees under the blanket, and turns onto her side, in obvious pain. She opens her mouth and gasps for air.

"I think," said Cohen, whose anger at W. R. Grace is intense, "that I would rather have mesothelioma than asbestosis. At least with mesothelioma it is over quickly."

8

JUSTICE DENIED

"I went to see Dr. Whitehouse in Spokane about six years ago, and he told me I had about five years, ten at the outside. I was driving back to Libby and all of the sudden it hit me and I had to pull off the side of the highway. Norita asked me what was wrong and I said, 'By God, you know something, I just got a death sentence.'"

—Les Skramstad

By the early 1990s, legal suits against asbestos companies had become commonplace, but no one had yet put the pieces of the puzzle together in Libby. W. R. Grace was already being hit with lawsuits over its Monokote product, but because asbestos wasn't an official ingredient of vermiculite, it didn't appear on the legal landscape as a target for plaintiff lawyers. Many Libby residents noticed that a large number of their neighbors seemed to be getting sick with bronchial problems, but Grace officials and the mine managers had done an effective job keeping a lid on the "tremolite problem." That lid may have stayed on for years had it not been for the Libby troublemakers.

"It had taken me a long time to get over the anger I felt when

131

Dad died," Gayla Benefield said. "The hurt in his eyes—he knew
they had killed him—is something I can never forget. Then, when
Mom got sick, I started suspecting something was really wrong. We
knew the miners ran a risk with the dust, but why did Mom have the
same symptoms? The sicker she got, the more I believed that Grace
and the mine was behind it."

Doing some investigating on her own, Benefield began to believe that even though the company knew her father was sick, they
put him back to work in the dusty, dry mill. "To me, that was
murder," she said. "They were trying to work him until he dropped
dead in his tracks. I thought, 'Okay, you bastards, you killed him.'"

Watching her mother turn from an optimistic, fun-loving
person into a sallow, pain-wracked, and bitter woman reopened
Benefield's deep reservoir of anger against the company. While she
tried to provide small comforts for her mother, there was nothing
anyone could do to keep Margaret Vatland from slowly suffocating.

Upon her mother's death in 1996, Benefield's sole focus became carrying out her promise. She would "get the bastards" no
matter what it took. The preposterous nature of the idea that a blue-
collar housewife from a dusty little town in a remote corner of Montana could stand up to a company run by a multimillionaire tycoon
who rubbed elbows and traded favors with popes, presidents, po-
tentates, and CIA directors never entered Benefield's mind. She was
a woman on a mission.

Les Skramstad is a cowboy at heart. He would have been happy
riding the range all his life, but cowboying didn't pay enough to support a family, so he took a job at the Zonolite mine instead. He was
a bagger at the mine, which meant he helped fill up to three hundred bags a day of whatever material was in the hopper. Sometimes
it was pure asbestos.

Skramstad started coughing in 1971, and he never stopped. "I just thought I had a chronic case of bronchitis," he said. "At one point the [operators of the mine] sent me over to a doctor in Seattle to see what was wrong. I remember he looked me right in the eye and said, 'What do you want me to say? You've got asbestosis.' I didn't have any idea what that was. I was never sent to that doctor again."

In 1996, long after Skramstad left the mine, Norita urged him to make the four-hour drive to Spokane see Dr. Alan Whitehouse, who had treated a few of their friends. When they arrived at White-house's eastern Spokane office, the doctor said, "You're from Libby. Well, I know why you are here."

Like the doctor in Seattle, Dr. Whitehouse diagnosed Skram-stad with asbestosis. This time, Skramstad understood the serious-ness of the disease and how he got it: the mine dust. The dust that the mine operators told him and everyone else was harmless. It was a monstrous lie. The dust was slowly killing him, and there wasn't anything anybody could do about it.

Quiet and easygoing by nature, Skramstad was more at home playing country music with his band, a feather in his cap, than he was sitting in a courtroom surrounded by lawyers in suits and ties. But the more he thought about it, the more he was convinced that the owners of the mine were wrong. They should have told him and the others and let them make up their own minds about working at the mines. He also knew that he would probably face es-calating medical costs as his condition worsened.

He had heard of other miners who had brought lawsuits against W. R. Grace, but he had never heard of any of them going to trial. In fact, Grace had settled them all out of court. With each set-tlement came a gag order on the plaintiff. They could have the money if they agreed not to talk about their case or the amount of the settlement. The confidentiality agreement on each settlement effectively kept the issue out of the newspapers and, more important, out of neighborhood conversations, which was the fastest method of mass communication in Libby.

But Skramstad was angry. He was angry that he was sick, angry that the company hadn't told him about the dangers of the asbestos dust, and angry that he had trouble getting enough breath to sing and play in his band. Calling a lawyer, he said he wanted to sue W. R. Grace.

The Skramstad case was the first to go to trial in Libby over the asbestos contamination that occurred at the Zonolite mine. Presiding over the case was a new judge in Libby, Michael Prezeau. Prezeau had been appointed to the bench in 1995 by Jim Racicot's cousin, Montana's Republican governor, Marc Racicot. The choice of Prezeau as presiding judge was an interesting one. His position prior to being appointed to the Libby bench was as a staff lawyer in a Missoula law firm that had represented Grace in several prior claims. Prezeau knew Marc Racicot from the early 1970s, when they had become friends in law school.

Skramstad's trial lasted two weeks. One of the exhibits the attorneys brought in was a large whiteboard that showed the medical arc of the rest of his life. It showed just when doctors expected him to sicken even further and die. Later, on the witness stand, he answered questions about his work at the mine. He was asked about his state of mind since he had been diagnosed with a terminal illness. He answered that he was suffering from periodic bouts of severe depression.

"The depression comes pretty regular," he testified.

"And what, do you think, that is attributable to?" the attorney asked.

"Lack of air," he answered.

At the end of the final week of the trial, Skramstad, Norita, and Benefield waited together to hear the jury's verdict. No newspaper reporters attended the trial and no one else was present except the lawyers. Skramstad was not optimistic. It seemed to him that the case had been tilted toward Grace.

Finally, the jury filed back into the room. They had a verdict. Skramstad sat, waiting for the bad news. He was shocked when the jury announced it had ruled in his favor and he was awarded $660,000. At first, the amount seemed like a fortune, but once his attorneys took their cut, plus expenses, he realized it would just be enough to cover his medical expenses before he died. At least he had won, though. The Zonolite mine was going to finally pay something for what it had done.

But the process was far from over. The Grace attorneys filed a brief with Judge Prezeau, who had to rule on the issue before the case could even be appealed. A year later, the judge had still not made a ruling. Desperate for money and afraid of the loophole in the Montana law that put no time limit on the judge's ruling, Skramstad told his attorneys to settle the case. He agreed to receive far less than the jury's award, and he felt the system had failed him once again.

It was years later before a journalist would question Prezeau about the Skramstad case. An unassuming, personable man, Prezeau turned away from the question with anguish on his face. "That was a tough one," he finally said. "It was complicated and . . ." He left the sentence unfinished. Prezeau then took several steps across the room, paused, and turned back again. "I can tell you I didn't delay the case intentionally," he said in a quiet voice. "It was terribly contentious. Every issue was subject to briefing battles and oral arguments. Both sides had dedicated troops working the file. It was just an incredibly slow process."

Talk of Prezeau's possible conflict of interest still lingers in some corners of Libby, but his veracity has never been questioned by anyone in an official position. Although his firm worked for Grace, he said he never worked on any cases involving the company, nor did he try to hide his past employment. He insisted that as a judge, he was impartial and had offered to recuse himself in trials involving Grace, but no plaintiff attorney ever asked him to do so. Skramstad, however, remains full of questions.

The day the settlement was completed was the worst day of Skramstad's life. A few moments prior to the completion of the deal, his wife, Norita, and their son, Brent, came back from the doctor. They had both just been diagnosed with asbestosis. He sat through the final settlement hearing in a daze. He was not allowed to say anything about his family. The Zonolite mine had won again.

During the Skramstad trial and a few that followed, the story of the Zonolite mine began to unfold. The 1959 study by the Zonolite Company, which sold the mine to Grace in 1963, that showed the high number of chest abnormalities in worker X rays; the years of constant warnings from the state of toxic air conditions at the mine; the intracompany memos from Grace officials warning against publicizing the dangerous work conditions and their bold acknowledgments that the vermiculite contained lethal amounts of tremolite (even as they donated the contaminated mine tailings for the construction of the high school running track); and their insistence in calling it "dust" rather than asbestos in public documents—all were revealed in the court cases.

At least seventy other cases were filed during a short time, and pretrial discoveries revealed that Grace officials had learned their strategy well from Johns-Manville.

One intracompany memo that was introduced into evidence, written by H. A. Eschenbach, director of Health, Safety, and Toxicology for Grace at the company's Massachusetts headquarters, dated June 5, 1972, suggests that Grace officials clearly knew that tremolite was carcinogenic. Eschenbach wrote:

> *During the week of May 15, I attended the annual conference of the American Industrial Hygiene Association. Many of the papers presented there concerned asbestos. Also, the monthly American Medical Association publication . . . has several asbestos related articles. These sources show that while most research involves chrysotile (Canadian asbestos) many of those involved with asbestos, naturally including Johns-Manville, believe that crocidolite is the 'bad actor.' . . . One observation of interest is that Libby tremolite and South African crocidolite appear to be identical. . . . One paper indicated that crocidolite is 5–10 [times] more carcinogenic than chrysotile. No one has had anything to say about tremolite and apparently no one is particularly interested at this time. However, the . . . similarity of crocidolite and tremolite is bound to eventually be of interest to someone and the obvious superficial conclusions could be less than desirable from our viewpoint. Unfortunately, there is little information available to refute any such allegation.*

In 1982, the company did an analysis of raw vermiculite ore in Libby. It revealed tremolite asbestos contamination in the range of from 21 to 26 percent. Despite the fact that Grace clearly knew that the vermiculite from its mine was contaminated with tremolite, which was "identical" to the "bad actor" crocidolite, Eschenbach wrote this to government regulators on March 24, 1983: "Finally we wish to emphasize that we have no reason to believe there is any risk associated with the current uses of Libby vermiculite-products."

The idea put forth early that Grace managers did not know about the dangers of asbestos was exploded by a series of documents, including X rays of the men that the company took that showed decades of highly elevated numbers of lung abnormalities. Included in evidence were the original 1959 X-ray studies and the fact that the results of this and other studies were never shared with the workers.

In addition, the number of warnings and studies done by Ben Wake for the State of Montana were introduced into evidence, as was the incendiary confidential 1967 intracompany memo that stated the company was aware that people were "contracting the disease in the yard or in fact at any point where a dust condition may exist." For the next twenty years after that memo was written, Grace would help spread vermiculite tailings, or the waste rock left over from the mining operation—which often had a much higher concentration of tremolite than did the deadly vermiculite itself—throughout the community.

A series of letters in 1979 between Eschenbach and Dr. Richard Irons of the Kootenai Clinic in Libby further underscored Grace's knowledge of the asbestos dangers. Dr. Irons, a doctor of internal medicine who worked for Dr. Brad Black at the clinic, made several overtures to Eschenbach regarding an occupational disease study he wanted to do at the mine. Dr. Irons was convinced that the risks at the mine were highly elevated, and he leaned on the Grace managers to purchase expensive medical equipment to conduct the study. In a March 19, 1979, letter to mine manager Earl Lovick, Dr. Irons spelled out the problems facing the workers.

"The documented pathologic effects of asbestos exposure in man include diffuse interstitial fibrosis [asbestosis], bronchial carcinoma, laryngeal cancer, malignant mesothelioma of the lung and abdominal peritoneum, [and] gastrointestinal cancers. . . . Finally, any attempt to consider risks to the workers must also extend to include their families and the community."

Lovick and Eschenbach parried with Dr. Irons while ridiculing him in intraoffice memos. "In summary, I think that Irons sees himself as the Selikoff of the tremolite world and Libby Hospital as the Mt. Sinai of the west," wrote Eschenbach.

When Dr. Irons threatened to do the study without the help of Grace managers, Eschenbach wrote to the managers at the mine that: "I think [Irons's] latest letter more or less puts his position on the line. We either play the game his way or he is going to blow the whistle."

Dr. Irons never did the study. Some time later, he left Libby, and the Libby Clinic never pressed the issue further.

The attitude of containment by the Grace managers emerged several times in the documents. An August 30, 1972, intracompany memo stated that a purchase order for fifty "Asbestos Warning Signs" had been signed by company managers. The signs were designed to comply with OSHA regulations. The memo stated, however, that use of the signs had to undergo review because "the introduction of the signs into the plants will present serious people problems, and this will require extreme care." None of the former mine workers can remember ever seeing any warning signs at the mine or the mill.

An internal memo from Grace executive O. F. Stewart to a mid-manager, dated February 29, 1972, showed how hard the company worked to keep a lid on the "tremolite problem" at Libby. Stewart was angry over an invitation sent to a representative of an asbestos company in Tacoma, Washington, who had expressed an interest in visiting the Libby mine to study the asbestos ore.

"Mr. Vining and I are getting quite concerned . . . about our people not following orders," Stewart wrote. "The Libby mine and mill is closed to visitors. Only those salesmen, etc., required to carry on daily business are to be allowed on the property without proper clearance. . . . You should not have discussed the asbestos with this man, but referred him to a higher authority. I would like a written explanation of your conversation. . . . The point I am trying to get across is that our present policy is to tell no one anything, no visitors, or discussion of our operations, period."

On March 30, 1977, an intracompany memo from Eschenbach put a halt on another proposed epidemiological study. "I believe that the results of a study of this nature would become public knowledge within a relatively short period of time regardless of confidentiality agreements," the memo stated. "If we are not prepared to deal with that situation, I would advise against proceeding."

In Michael Brown's documentary *Dust to Dust*, Lovick, by then a silver-haired man in his seventies, is shown being grilled by a plaintiff's attorney regarding the company's knowledge of the asbestos contamination at the mine. The deposition took place in the late 1990s, nearly a decade after Lovick retired. He had worked at the mine for thirty years, much of that time as the executive manager.

Lovick appeared a terribly nervous and broken man as he testified openly that the management did not tell the miners about the true dangers of the asbestos.

> *Q: What is your understanding of what asbestosis is?*
> *Lovick: My understanding is it is a disease of the lungs.*
>
> *Q: To your knowledge, have X workers at Zonolite died of it?*
> *Lovick: To my knowledge, X workers have died and one of the causes of death is asbestosis. I don't recall if the death*

certificates said it was a primary cause but it would have been a contributing factor.

Q: Were some of these people friends of yours?
Lovick: *Yes sir.*

Q: As of 1956, the company knew there was asbestos in the dust. Is that correct?
Lovick: *Yes sir, I would agree with that.*

Q: As of 1956, did Zonolite do anything to inform the employees what asbestosis was?
Lovick: *Not that I recall, no sir.*

Q: And the company also knew that asbestosis is from inhaling asbestos dust. Correct?
Lovick: *Yes sir.*

Q: And the company also knew there were workers at Zonolite who were inhaling asbestos dust. Correct?
Lovick: *Yes sir.*

Soon after her mother died, Benefield also filed suit against W. R. Grace. "People thought I was a crazy woman," she said, "but I knew what the company had done. It was a nightmare come true."

Benefield was living on a mountain of anger. The mine had killed both her parents and a number of her friends, but so far everyone filing suit against Grace had settled before going to trial. The gag orders kept the story from getting out, and no one at Grace was being forced to admit that they had done anything wrong.

It was apparent to Benefield that the government was not going to step in and bring Grace to justice, so the legal suit she filed with her sister would have to do. The Grace attorneys immediately came up with a settlement offer for ten thousand dollars. Benefield felt like spitting in their faces. Her attorneys prepared for trial. Near the time the trial was to begin, the Grace attorneys, convinced that Benefield's case was strong, came back with another offer. This time more than $600,000 was put on the table, along with something Benefield wanted more than anything—an apology from the company.

It seemed like a reasonable offer. For Benefield, there was only one final question.

"Can I post the results of this settlement on the Internet?" she asked.

The Grace attorneys reacted as if they had just tasted spoiled milk. They insisted the settlement must contain a gag order, just like all the rest. Benefield and her sister could have the money, but they couldn't talk about the case to anyone.

The others in the case urged Benefield to take the deal. They were afraid Grace would take their substantial offer off the table at any moment. "I told the Grace attorneys to take the money and shove it," said Benefield. "I didn't feel that making the company pay what was, to them, an insignificant amount was keeping my promise to my mother. There was no way they would pay the least bit of attention to us. I wanted to make what they did public. I wanted a trial where it would all come out and the community and the world would realize what they had done."

Benefield got her wish. The case went to trial, and the Grace offer left the table. The money in the settlement offer would have made a huge difference to Benefield and her family. She knew the risk she was taking. She sat through most of the Skramstad trial and knew he had clearly won his case. Yet there always seemed to be technicalities, always a reason that people—especially people who weren't rich or powerful—never seemed to receive full justice. She knew that even if she won, she might not see as much money as Grace had already offered. But Benefield had made up her mind. She wasn't about to let Grace buy her silence.

As the trial finally began in the late fall of 1998, an odd thought occurred to Benefield. It was getting so that in Libby, she knew more people in the cemetery than she knew in the town. That thought, plus the mental images she kept of her mother and father suffering the final stages of their diseases, strengthened her resolve. The Grace attorneys were powerful men who intimidated most of those around them, but Benefield didn't fear them. She believed the company had already done all the damage it could in her life. Her anger helped carry her through the pressures of the trial.

Some of the most telling testimony in the trial came from Dr. David Egilman, the asbestos expert from Brown University. Dr. Egilman testified that the 92 percent worker disease rate revealed among twenty-year workers at the mine was "the highest reported rate of lung disease in any group of workers exposed to an asbestos form of mineral that I've seen."

Dr. Egilman was also asked why it was so critical that Grace did not properly give the workers a full appreciation of the asbestos risk. He responded by saying that asbestos has no "onion" properties—you can't smell, see, touch, or taste fibers in the air. "If there was a snowstorm of asbestos in this room now, we would feel fine, and not only would we feel fine today, but we'd feel fine tomorrow and the next day," he testified. "It wouldn't make you itch like fiberglass. It wouldn't irritate your nose. It wouldn't make your vision blurry. It wouldn't smell bad. Most of it looks relatively clean-looking, white.

"So, your normal five senses don't tell you it's dangerous," he added. "In fact, your normal senses and your experience either. You can't see it, and it doesn't make you feel bad, and it takes a long time before it makes you feel bad. So you can go back into that snow-storm every day, month after month, potentially year after year and you feel fine. So your common sense tells you, 'This isn't so bad. I'm working. I'm not short of breath. My nose doesn't irritate me. It doesn't bother my skin.' It's a hidden hazard, and, in fact, it takes so little of it to make you sick, so it is literally hidden and figuratively hidden, and the only way to know about it and deal with it is to tell people about it and tell them to take precautions."

The jury deliberations did not take long. Benefield's spirits soared as the judgment was announced in her favor, but a short time later they plunged again as the award was announced. Grace was ordered to pay Benefield and her sister a total of $250,000—less than half of the settlement offer. After attorneys' fees and expenses, and after she split the net figure with her sister, Benefield's share came to $67,000. "So that is what my mother's life was worth," she thought. Still, she didn't regret her decision to reject the gag order. Her children had backed her in the decision to reject the settlement offer, and she knew she had set the right example for them by not selling out to Grace. Most important of all, now the information was public. She felt that Grace was finally exposed for what it was: a cutthroat corporation that cared far more for profits than for people's lives. Finally, Benefield thought, the world would realize what Grace had done to the people of Libby.

The days went by after the trial, however, and she heard no mention of it anywhere. Finally, three weeks later, the local paper ran a small story on the inside pages. Meanwhile, it ran a large, front-page story lauding Lovick for his contributions to the community. Benefield was devastated. It seemed that W. R. Grace had won again.

9

1980–2002: POLITICAL FAILURES

Of all the missed opportunities in the last half of the twentieth century to rid America of the plague of asbestos, none were more poignant than the unfortunate legal and political decisions that were made in 1991. Two decades earlier, the fledgling EPA had become increasingly concerned about the harmful health effects of asbestos. The large body of scientific and medical evidence, crowned by the work of Dr. Selikoff, had long proved conclusively that asbestos exposure was a serious health problem. By the late 1970s, the EPA, taking its charter to protect the health of Americans seriously, was working on a long-range asbestos phaseout ban. The ambitious project soon ran into a number of roadblocks, including objections from the Office of Management and Budget and an avalanche of demands for reviews by makers and users of asbestos products.

Ultimately, it took the EPA ten years and ten million dollars to design and implement the ban. To its credit, the EPA met every challenge, and on July 6, 1989, William K. Reilly, the administrator of the agency, formally announced that the manufacture and sale of an estimated 84 percent of asbestos products in the United States—including brake linings, roofing, pipe, tile, and insulation—would be prohibited. The ban was also designed to stop the export of asbestos products, which Reilly said left "a terrible legacy of dead, dying and crippled."

The ban came at a time when asbestos use had already dropped in the United States from 560,000 metric tons in 1979 to 55,000 metric tons in 1989, due in large part to "voluntary" cutbacks by asbestos manufacturers. In truth, these cutbacks were due to two factors, neither of them stemming from the benevolence of the industry. First, the asbestos companies were already facing tens of thousands of legal suits by plaintiffs with asbestos-related diseases. The plaintiff lawyers were finally doing what federal regulators had failed to do for sixty years: motivate the manufacturers to find alternatives to asbestos. Second, the federal government, primarily under the Jimmy Carter administration, actually did put some pressure on manufacturers to pull the asbestos out of their products.

In 1979, an analysis of the fiber emission levels of handheld hair dryers—nearly all of which contained asbestos as a heat shield insulator—was done for the U.S. Consumer Product Safety Commission (CPSC) by Dr. William J. Nicholson of the Environmental Sciences Laboratory at Mount Sinai Hospital. Nicholson found that the hair dryers emitted "considerable quantities" of asbestos each time they were used. "The fiber concentrations in the effluent of some dryers exceeded the highest we have measured in eight years of surveillance of environmental asbestos contamination," Nicholson said.

Faced with such damning evidence, the thirty-seven companies that shared the market of the more than twelve million handheld asbestos-containing dryers manufactured or sold in the United States agreed to cease production and distribution of their products. Similar "voluntary" bans were placed on asbestos paper products, beauty salon hair dryers, and some children's toys, such as Milton Bradley's Fibro-Clay, a school art-modeling compound used to make papier-mâché.

The CPSC had already approved a ban on consumer patching

compounds and artificial fireplace ash containing asbestos in 1977. In general, the CPSC took a more aggressive stance against all potential cancer-causing substances found in consumer products under President Carter, asbestos being one of them. In 1980, the agency moved to require twelve hundred U.S. corporations to provide information regarding their use of asbestos in products. Most of these efforts were halted during the Reagan administration. (In an ironic twist, when the agency added staff under President Clinton, it was forced to relocate its headquarters because asbestos insulation in the walls and ceilings of the old headquarters prevented expansion and renovation.)

Despite these "voluntary" cutback efforts by manufacturers, thousands of asbestos products were still on the market in the late 1980s, and the EPA felt strongly that a federal ban was the only effective way to stop the massive exposures that were occurring nationwide. The ban called for roofing and flooring felt, tile, and clothing made from asbestos to be prohibited by 1990. The second stage of the ban would have eliminated about 20 percent of the asbestos products on the market by 1993, including brake linings, transmission components, clutch facings, and other friction and gasket materials. The final stage called for the prohibition of asbestos in pipes, shingles, brake blocks, paper, and most other products with asbestos as an ingredient.

The ban was hailed by most health experts, although some felt it did not go far enough. The intrusion of international politics could be felt in the hedging done at the news conference that Reilly held to announce the ban. "This action should not be seen as a signal to other nations, especially developing nations, that use of these products should be discontinued," Reilly said. The reference was aimed primarily at trying to placate the Canadian government, one of the world's largest asbestos exporters. Political expediency, in this case, overwhelmed the obvious and blatant hypocrisy of the double standard. Nevertheless, the domestic ban marked the first definitive action ever taken in the United States to halt the additional exposure of tens of thousands of Americans.

The Asbestos Information Association of North America, which at the time represented an estimated twenty Canadian and U.S. asbestos companies, called the rules "draconian." The association reacted with incredulity, stating that such a ban would force the companies to stop producing asbestos products, which, of course, is exactly what the EPA hoped to do. A short time later, a consortium of asbestos companies from the U.S. and Canada filed suit to have the ban overturned.

The case was heard in 1991 by the 5th Circuit Court of Appeals in New Orleans. The three-judge appellate court was presented evidence that after reviewing more than a hundred studies of asbestos, and having taken testimony in several public meetings, the EPA concluded, "Asbestos is a potential carcinogen at all levels of exposure."

In the end, however, the case was decided less on the relative merits of the scientific and health studies than on a technicality. The judges ruled in favor of the asbestos companies, blaming the EPA for "its failure to give adequate weight to statutory language requiring it to promulgate the least burdensome, reasonable regulation required to protect the environment adequately." The appellate court did uphold a prohibition against the sale of newly designed asbestos products, but the more than three thousand products already on the market remained unregulated.

EPA employees were stunned. Given that the agency had already determined that asbestos caused cancer at all levels of exposure, how could the judges find that there was a regulation that would be "less burdensome" than the phaseout ban and still protect American lives? To many observers, the decision defied logic.

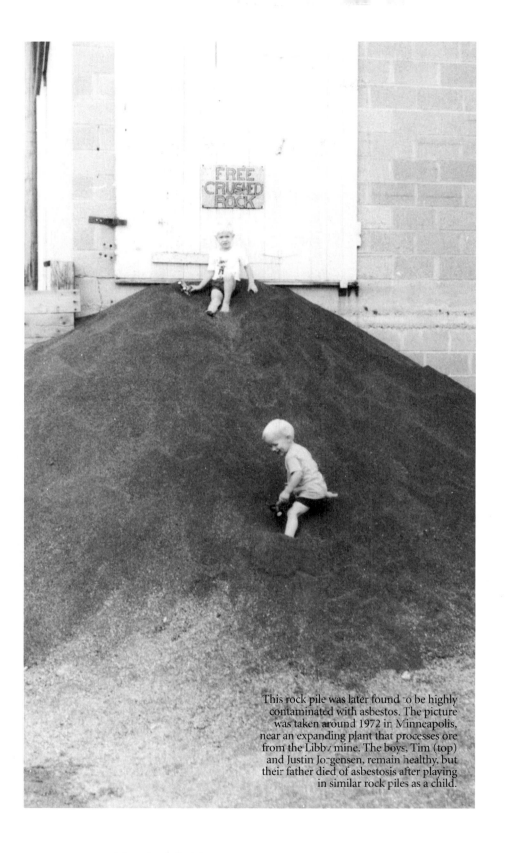

This rock pile was later found to be highly contaminated with asbestos. The picture was taken around 1972 in Minneapolis, near an expanding plant that processes ore from the Libby mine. The boys, Tim (top) and Justin Jorgensen, remain healthy, but their father died of asbestosis after playing in similar rock piles as a child.

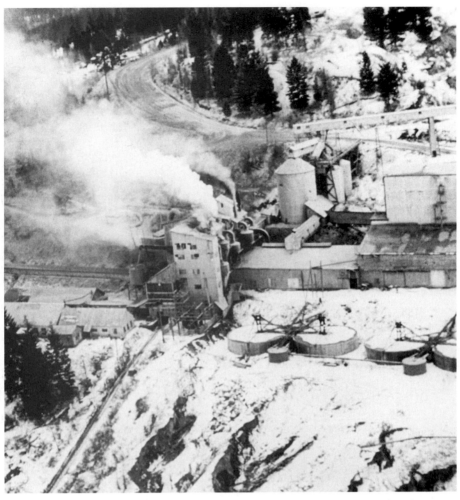

Smoke pours out of the vermiculite mill north of Libby, Montana. The mill was closed in 1990.

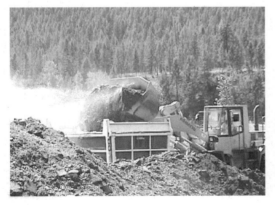

EPA crews remove asbestos-contaminated soils from the site of the old screening plant. Easter sunrise services for the town were held near here on the banks of the Kootenai River before the contamination was discovered.

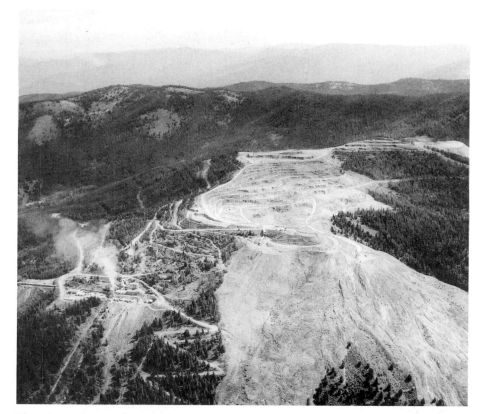

The mine at the top of Vermiculite Mountain. Waste rock, which was pushed over the edge of the mountain and can be seen in the foreground, was used to build the running tracks at Libby High School and Libby Middle School.

High-pressure hoses were used to clean the EPA trucks before they left the contaminated screening plant site in Libby. Billions of microscopic asbestos fibers can cling to the dirt and mud on the trucks and, if not washed off, can contaminate roadways.

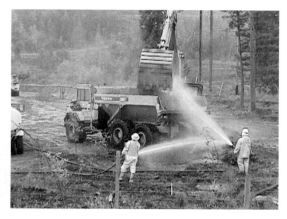

The baseball fields in Libby were contaminated with asbestos for decades. The expanding plant in the background spewed fibers almost daily (photo circa 1955).

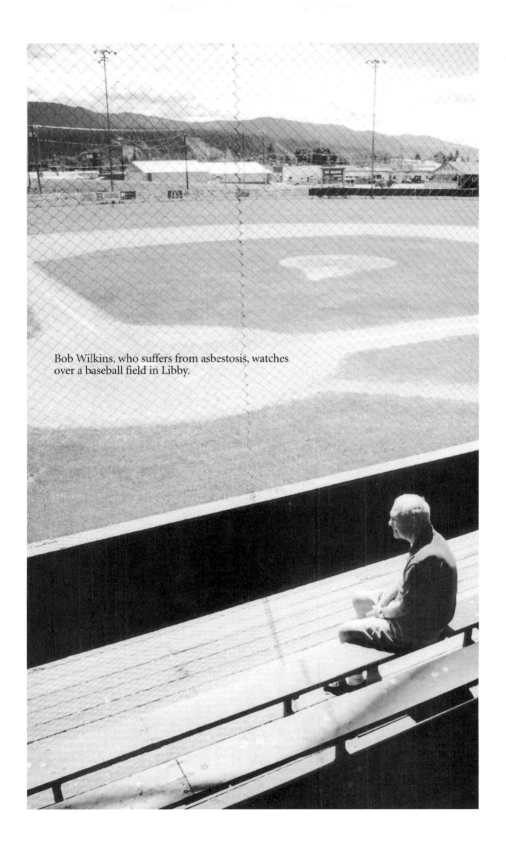

Bob Wilkins, who suffers from asbestosis, watches over a baseball field in Libby.

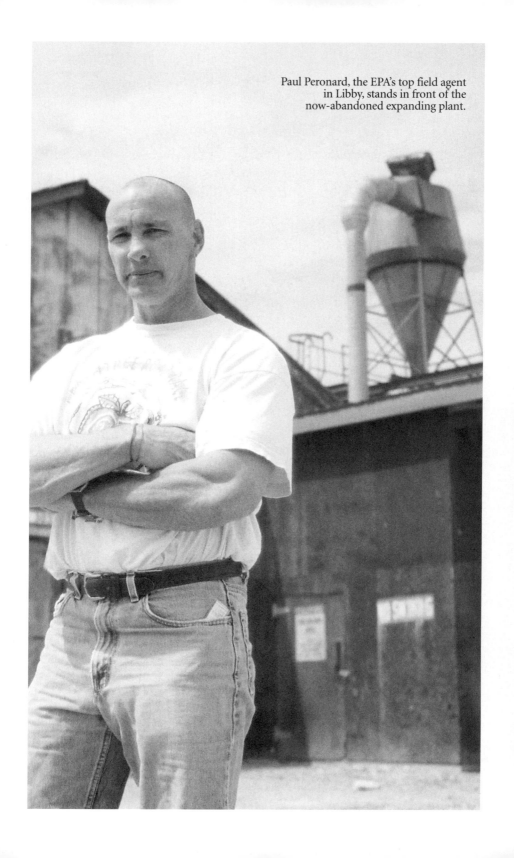

Paul Peronard, the EPA's top field agent in Libby, stands in front of the now-abandoned expanding plant.

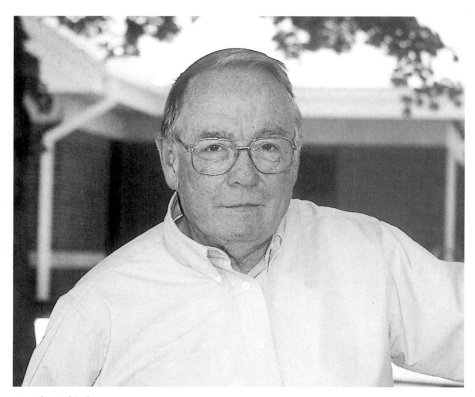

Dr. Alan Whitehouse

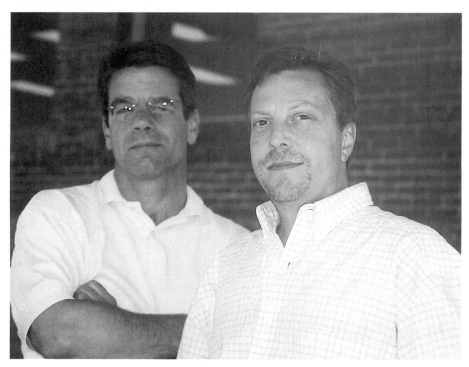

Chris Weis (l) and Dr. Aubrey Miller

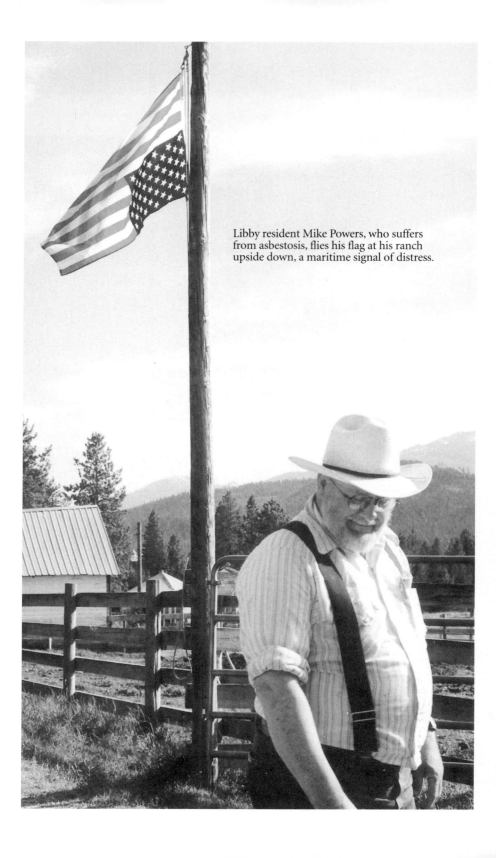

Libby resident Mike Powers, who suffers from asbestosis, flies his flag at his ranch upside down, a maritime signal of distress.

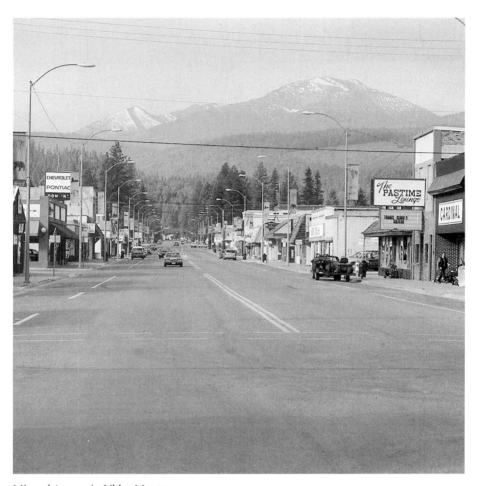

Mineral Avenue in Libby, Montana

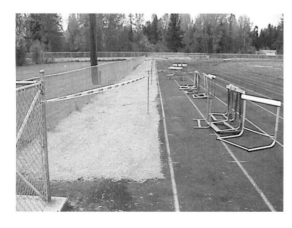

The high school running track in Libby was originally made from asbestos-contaminated tailings.

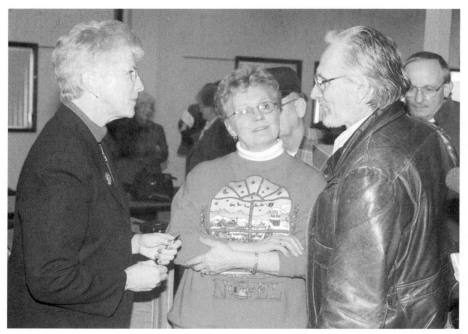

Gayla Benefield (c) and Les Skramstad (r) confer with Montana governor Judy Martz.

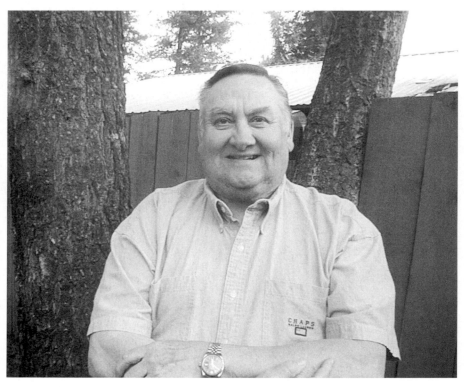

Jim Racicot

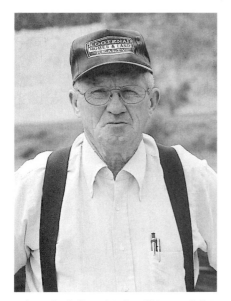
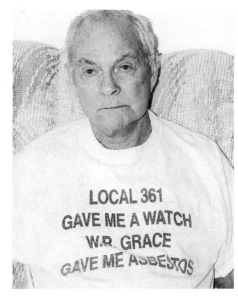

Bob Dedrick (l) and Bob Wilkins are fighting to save their town. Both suffer from asbestos-caused disease.

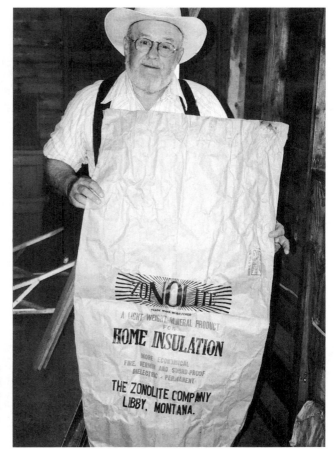

Libby resident Mike Powers holds a Zonolite Insulation bag. The product was shipped nationwide.

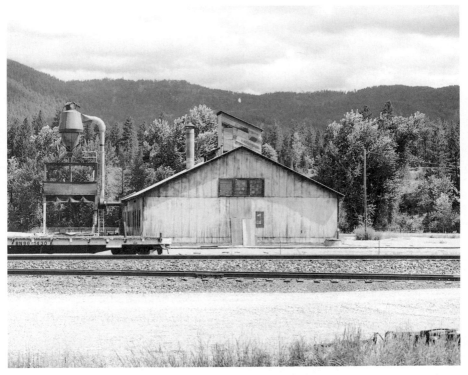

This building was part of the expanding plant that processed contaminated ore. For several decades, it was surrounded by baseball fields.

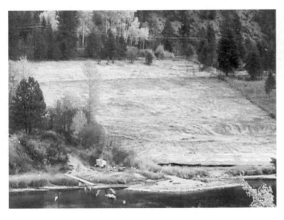

Site of W. R. Grace's former screening plant on the Kootenai River that was razed and cleaned to the subsoil level by the EPA.

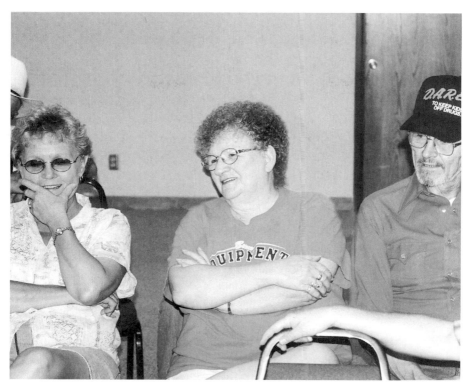

Gayla Benefield (l), Norita Skramstad, and Les Skramstad (r), three Libby "troublemakers"

Rainy Creek Road, which led
to the Libby mine, was so
contaminated it had to be
cleaned and paved by the EPA.

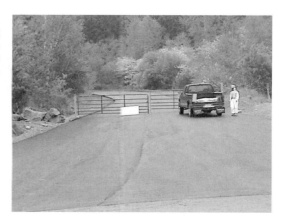

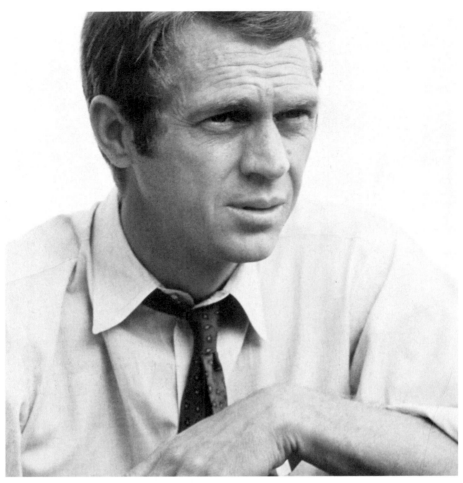

Actor Steve McQueen died from asbestos poisoning at age fifty.

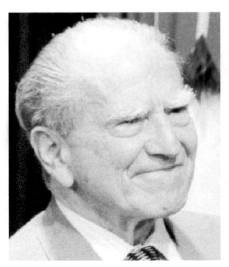

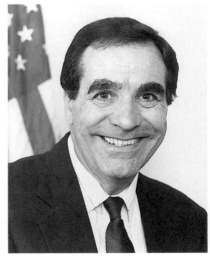

Asbestos victims Navy admiral Elmo Zumwalt (l) and Minnesota Congressman Bruce Vento

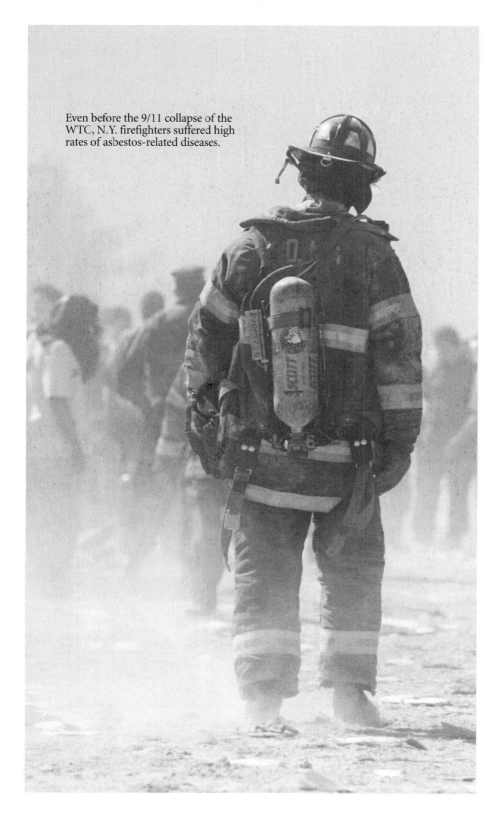

Even before the 9/11 collapse of the
WTC, N.Y. firefighters suffered high
rates of asbestos-related diseases.

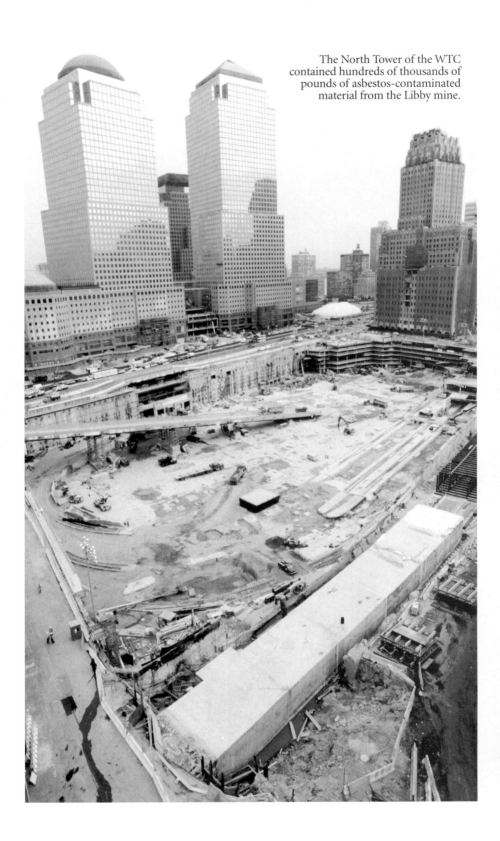

The North Tower of the WTC contained hundreds of thousands of pounds of asbestos-contaminated material from the Libby mine.

In overturning the ban, however, the court also found that the EPA had not done enough homework in terms of determining whether there were adequate and safer alternatives that could be substituted for the asbestos in the various products. This was a more logical point, but the feeling within the EPA was strong that the appellate court's ruling would be overturned if the case was appealed to the Supreme Court.

The ban, however, died a quiet and ignominious death. The Bush Sr. administration refused to allow the EPA to address the "faulty" alternatives section of its brief, nor would it allow the case to be appealed. The result was the demolition of ten years of work by the EPA, total confusion on the part of the public regarding the legality of asbestos, and a green light given by the government to the asbestos companies to continue to market their products with little governmental regulation.

Of all the ironies in the asbestos story, perhaps the darkest can be found in the words used by the 5th Appellate Court to describe the EPA ban. Quoting the asbestos industry lawyers, the court referred to the ban as the "death penalty alternative" because it was considered the most burdensome of all the possible options for regulating the asbestos industry. It was curious language given the staggering toll on human life that asbestos had already exacted.

The asbestos lobby included some of the wealthiest and most powerful companies in the world. Aside from Grace and Johns-Manville, they included Raybestos-Manhattan, Owens Corning, Unarco, Union Carbide, Philip Carey Manufacturing, National Gypsum, GAF Materials, Eagle-Picher, the Keene Corporation, and dozens of smaller companies. Few politicians dared take on the asbestos Goliath. Other than the EPA's aborted ban, there were few other serious political efforts to protect asbestos workers or consumers.

The depth to which some of the industry leaders were tied to the innermost dealings of America's top politicians can be seen in the life and times of Peter Grace. Few men in any industry were more entangled in the foreign affairs of the U.S. government than the man who once said that his two hobbies were "economics and anticommunism."

Grace was a well-connected and powerful man. His position as head of a major corporate power, multimillion-dollar personal fortune, worldwide connections, and kinetic personality made him an unpredictable and uncontrollable force that sometimes frightened his own allies. He continually made the New York Catholic Church circles nervous with his constant schemes to get the church involved with what many felt were overtly political actions. He was a major rainmaker for the Catholic Church, but his phenomenal fundraising efforts were offset by fears he would someday drag it into a political scandal. Author Penny Lernoux, in her book *People of God: The Struggle for World Catholicism* (Viking, 1989), described Grace as "high-handed, ambitious and frenetically busy." He was abrupt with employees and worked sixteen to eighteen hours a day, giving that as the reason he never married. Grace always wore two watches, one with the local time wherever he happened to be, the other with the time back in New York headquarters. He sometimes dictated to two secretaries at a time, and he often wore a gun in his belt—which he liked to display along with his thirty-four-inch waist, "one of his many vanities," wrote Lernoux.

Grace was, without question, a superb businessman. During his forty-seven years at the helm of his grandfather's company, he turned it from a midlevel business with $12 million in annual sales to a world power generating more than $5 billion in revenue in the mid-1980s. He led Grace longer than any other head of a major U.S. company in the last half of the twentieth century. His official company bio always proudly mentioned that after graduation from Yale in 1936, he started in the company's mailroom and worked his way up to chairman of the board. The fact that his grandfather and father preceded him in that position may, of course, have played a role in his ascendancy.

Profoundly religious, Grace was deeply involved with the Catholic Church. His personal résumé was impressive. He was the president of the Catholic Youth Organization of the Archdiocese of New York, a fervent supporter of the Boys Clubs of America, and he helped found the Covenant House for homeless boys and the Inner City Scholarship Fund. He advised cardinals and was a frequent visitor to the Vatican. Twenty-five universities gave him honorary degrees. He served President Dwight Eisenhower as a member of the International Advisory Board and put his name to a widely circulated report called "An Economic Program of the Americas." At the time, Grace was probably the nation's top expert on conducting business in Central America and South America. He ran the company with the same iron fist as his grandfather. W. R. Grace, who was given the nickname "the Pirate of Peru" by those who felt he may have been a bit heavy-handed with the local populace. The company was undeniably successful, however. Under Peter Grace, it would ultimately operate in more than a hundred countries.

In 1962, Grace worked with twenty-nine other top business executives to promote U.S. trade in Latin America as part of President Kennedy's Commerce Committee for the Alliance for Progress. The connection between the ultraconservative Grace and Kennedy might have seemed an odd one except for the fact that they may have been the two most powerful Catholics in the country in the early 1960s.

While his leadership of one of the world's largest companies gave Grace significant political clout, it may well have been the proverbial tip of the iceberg. Grace's story took an unexpected and almost surreal twist in the years following WWII, when he was selected to lead a U.S. arm of an elite Catholic organization called the Knights of Malta, officially titled the Sovereign Military Order of Malta. This exclusive organization is the modern version of a religious order that was established one thousand years ago to help care for the sick and poor. Later, it took on a military role as the organization played a major role in the defense of the Christian settlements in Palestine and Syria. The organization gained its modern name after the Catholics were driven from Palestine and ultimately settled on the island of Malta. Although closely aligned with the Vatican, the Knights of Malta, whose members include some of the world's most powerful figures, is autonomous in its worldwide dealings.

Grace, who viewed himself as a crusader and a religious knight, headed the most influential U.S. branch that was established by a group of powerful, conservative businessmen in the late 1920s, among them John Raskob, chairman of the board of General Motors. They were soon joined by John Farrell, president of U.S. Steel, and by Joseph P. Grace and Joseph Kennedy, whose sons would use the connection to work together to further their separate ambitions. At the time that Grace became president of the major U.S. branch, the membership also reportedly included William F. Buckley Jr., Valéry Giscard D'Estaing, General Alexander Haig, Walter Schellenburg, William Simon, William Clark, J. Edgar Hoover, Lee Iacocca, Senator Ted Kennedy, Thomas "Tip" O'Neill, Henry Luce, and Pat Buchanan.

Perhaps more tellingly, it also included Bill Donovan and Allen Dulles, who helped found the Central Intelligence Agency following WWII; John McCone, director of the CIA under Kennedy; and William Casey, the CIA director under Reagan. It also included honorary member Prescott Bush Jr., the brother of George Bush Sr., who would be involved with Grace in several other organizations and projects.

The Knights of Malta, despite members such as Kennedy and O'Neill, was a rigorously conservative organization. Although publicly it focused on raising millions of dollars to help the world's poor, it also actively supported conservative, anticommunist activities worldwide. Most of the vast contributions came from multinational corporations that, like the Vatican, feared and hated communism. It was that fear that may well have driven the fledgling CIA, and members of the Knights of Malta, into taking clandestine actions that historians have since strongly questioned.

The first was the organization's alleged involvement with helping to "cleanse" the records of Nazi scientists so they could enter the U.S. following WWII. Called Operation Paperclip, the strategy was to utilize these scientists in the Cold War against the Soviet Union and to aid American corporations.

Just exactly what the Knights of Malta's role in Operation Paperclip was interested many, but what is on record is the CIA's recruitment of high-ranking Nazi general Reinhard Gehlen, who ultimately ran the CIA's surveillance on the Soviet Union until the late 1960s. Gehlen, who ran the anti-Soviet spy ring for Adolf Hitler, reportedly stashed all the information he had on the Soviets in fifty-five-gallon drums when it became clear that Germany was losing the war. He buried the drums throughout the Alps and at the end of the war made a deal with American intelligence officers to give up the information in exchange for a position in what would become the CIA. This information, rumored for decades and written about in at least five books on the CIA, was officially released by the agency in the fall of 2000.

The CIA filed an affidavit in U.S. District Court "acknowledging an intelligence relationship with German General Reinhard

Gehlen that it has kept secret for 50 years. . . . The CIA's announcement marks the first acknowledgement by that agency that it had any relationship with Gehlen," a National Archives press release stated.

"Gehlen's network of agents in Europe—including many with Nazi backgrounds who were bailed out of prisoner of war camps by U.S. intelligence officers—was known as the Gehlen Organization and received millions of dollars in funding from the U.S. until 1956," the *New York Post* reported.

In 1948, the Knights of Malta awarded Gehlen, who was only four years removed from Hitler's headquarters, the Grand Cross of Honor for his work in fighting communism.

Decades later, the Grace-CIA connection made headlines again when the *Washington Post* broke a story in 1992 indicating that W. R. Grace was involved in an illegal money-funneling operation to fight communists in Nicaragua that was similar to the Iran-Contra scandal, but on a smaller scale. Grace officials denied any involvement.

By the late 1970s and throughout the 1980s, Peter Grace moved easily within the most powerful circles in the world. It was not unusual for him to appear publicly with both Democrats and Republicans, although his own politics were deeply conservative. On December 9, 1979, for example, he appeared on the dais with President Jimmy Carter and Senator Kennedy at a birthday dinner–Boston College fund-raiser for Tip O'Neill. He also served on an impressive number of policy-making bodies for foundations and boards ranging from Citicorp, Citibank, Ingersoll-Rand, Milliken & Company, and Kennecott Cooper to Magnavox, and he was a trustee of the Atlantic Mutual insurance company. Grace was also the chairman of Radio Free Europe/Radio Liberty Fund. He served on a number of organizations having political and humanistic goals in South America and Central America, including AmeriCares, a private, voluntary organization closely associated with the Knights of Malta. AmeriCares, a nonprofit disaster-relief program founded in 1975, distributes food and health supplies throughout the world, usually in unsettled areas where America is still fighting for influence, such as Central America, Lebanon, and Afghanistan. Other directors included former treasury secretary William Simon and Prescott Bush.

Privately, Grace was determined to move his company forward through diversification and the sale of its South American operations, which he concluded were too politically shaky for long-term business stability. He redirected the company away from shipping, cotton, and other Latin American products and concentrated on building a U.S. base by acquiring a number of small, specialty chemical companies. The Libby vermiculite mine fit perfectly into his plans. It was a cash cow and helped him purchase a number of smaller, diverse companies. Grace subsidiaries made packaging films, bags, and laminates and developed cracking catalysts to produce gasoline and other fuels. Zonolite and Monokote were "high-tech" products that pushed profits ever higher. The company also made container-sealing compounds that went into about four billion food and beverage bottles and cans annually. It operated restaurants and branched into home health care services and kidney dialysis services. Under Peter Grace, the old company his grandfather had started more than one hundred years before morphed into a diversified giant with tentacles that reached around the world.

Despite his high profile in government circles, Grace was not as well known to the American public as some of his counterparts, like Lee Iacocca. Most of Grace's products were sold to other industries rather than directly to the consumer, and there was no reason for the company or Grace to personally market his products on television as Iacocca did. The same was true for most asbestos company executives, who realized their relative anonymity served to help keep them from media and public scrutiny. Grace was best known during the early 1980s when he was appointed by President Reagan to head the task force on ways to reduce government spending. Its mission was to "work like tireless bloodhounds to root out government inefficiency and waste of tax dollars."

Grace took his charge seriously, and the task force quickly took on the official name of the Grace Commission. At the same time, he was flying practically nonstop around the country, galvanizing his friends in the oil, plastics, and chemical industries to recommend ways of cutting back on governmental regulations. In all, the Grace Commission produced some twenty-five hundred recommendations, many of which called for the trimming of the governmental budget for environmental and occupational safety regulations. The committee concluded its work with a report that contained a whopping twenty-one thousand pages.

Grace later boasted that the recommendations of his commission would have saved the government and corporations hundreds of billions of dollars. After the Congressional Budget Office and the General Accounting Office reviewed the recommendations, however, few were implemented.

In 1984, Grace, fired up from his crusade to trim the "fat" from government, founded a private, nonprofit organization called Citizens Against Government Waste. It was to be a privately run extension of the Grace Commission.

Of the multiplicity of tidy and untidy ironies in the asbestos story, Grace's obsession with governmental economic waste is perhaps the most colorful. In the end, the choice to continue manufacturing and marketing asbestos products with minimum public disclosure about the accompanying risks would prove to be perhaps the most expensive and avoidable mistake ever made by American corporate leaders. Not only will it ultimately cost the federal and state governments billions of dollars in court costs, health coverage, and a host of related regulatory and abatement costs, it ultimately bankrupted many of the companies themselves—including W. R. Grace.

As lawsuits pile up by the hundreds of thousands, Congress has been urged by both sides to provide legislation to handle the problem. Congress, in response, has been unwilling to provide a solution.

There have been a number of legislative attempts over the past few decades, but they have been so blatantly procorporation that the trial lawyers and unions have opposed them unanimously.

Vice President Dick Cheney, the CEO from 1995 to 2000 of the energy giant Halliburton Company, which faces asbestos litigation from the acquisition of a company that utilized asbestos in the past, was a major player in attempting to pass procorporate legislation before running for public office. During the Cheney years, Halliburton contributed more than $150,000 to congressional members. Since becoming vice president, Cheney has kept a low public profile regarding the asbestos industry.

One of the problems facing congressional members is the complicated set of medical issues surrounding asbestos. The pathology of asbestos-related diseases is complex, made more so by claims based on advocacy rather than science. The long latency period before the disease clearly presents itself opens the door to all manner of claims as to its "benign" nature. It has only been in the last few years that Congress has heard much testimony from scientists and doctors, and, most important, from the asbestos victims themselves.

One of the first to testify was Fred Biekkola, a sixty-seven-year-old retired mine worker from Michigan. Biekkola worked for thirty-one years in open-pit iron ore mines near L'Anse, a small Upper Peninsula community not far from Marquette on Lake Superior. The iron-mining operations used thousands of tons of asbestos in the kilns and crushers that helped process the ore. Biekkola was part of a crew that mixed the asbestos with heavy oil in fifty-five-gallon drums. The men were told that the huge amounts of dust present in the crushing operation were harmless.

"I was big and strong and like the rest of the guys. I thought I was Superman, that a little dust couldn't hurt me," said Biekkola, who now has an advanced case of asbestosis. "It wasn't long after we retired that guys started dying. Of the six guys I worked with, I went to five of their houses during the last two weeks of their lives and watched them die. We just didn't know."

Ellen Biekkola is still fiercely angry with the men at the local iron company she feels poisoned her husband. "They traded him a job for cancer," she said. "They make a fool of you, they laugh at you, they won't even admit there was asbestos there to this day. I don't know how you can ever beat them and their lawyers. If it was up to me, I would throw them all into the lake and drown them."

Her anger comes from a betrayal that came as a total surprise to the workers and their families. Ellen and Fred met at a Fourth of July parade in 1957 and fell in love. They were married two years later. Like most young couples, they dreamed of owning a house and raising their four children. Fred's job at the mines allowed them to pursue their dream. Today, the dream has turned into a nightmare.

"This is especially upsetting to our kids," said Ellen. "They worry about their dad and they are pretty angry at the mining companies. I'm angry too. What I don't understand is that for all those years Fred was the most loyal employee that company could ever want. He worked extra shifts whenever they asked, and sometimes he drove through snowstorms to get there. Tonight he has to go to the funeral home and eulogize one of his friends who just died from asbestosis. People are dying horrible deaths from asbestos all around this community, but even the local newspaper doesn't seem interested. *Asbestos*—when I hear that word it makes my hair stand on end."

In 2001, Fred was asked to testify before Congress during hearings called by Washington senator Patty Murray. The first words he spoke were simple and powerful. "Senators," Biekkola began, "they lied to us."

Despite her husband's testimony, Ellen remains dubious that anything will be done. "It's all about the ungodly dollar," she said. "I don't know how you stop it because it is such a big thing. Maybe there are answers, but I don't think you can trust our political system to find them. How can they justify allowing the sale of products that kill people? I'd like to ask every congressperson to answer that question."

10

A LEGAL RECKONING

If, by the 1980s, the media, the government, and the American populace did not yet grasp the full scope of the devastation and tragedy caused by the asbestos industry's strategy of concealment, plaintiff lawyers did. Their clients were growing by the thousands, and the evidence against the industry was becoming overwhelming. Plaintiff investigators were ripping the shroud off the industry's fifty-year cover-up by discovering memos like the one from the Johns-Manville medical director to J-M corporate headquarters, which addressed the growing problem of asbestosis among J-M workers: "The fibrosis of this disease is irreversible and permanent so that eventually compensation will be paid to each of these men," the memo stated. "But, as long as the man is not disabled it is felt that he should not be told of his condition so that he can live and work in peace and the company can benefit by his many years of experience."

To plaintiff attorneys, this kind of statement was like chum in the water. For whatever motivated them, the fact is, it was ultimately the hard work and persistence of a handful of plaintiff attorneys that helped curb the abuses of the asbestos industry, a job that should have been done by government regulators and lawmakers long before.

The first asbestos-product lawsuit was filed December 10, 1966, in Beaumont, Texas. The plaintiff, Claude Tomplait, an asbestos worker in Lake Charles, Louisiana, had been diagnosed with "pulmonary dust disease" and suffered from all the classic physical signs of asbestosis. The defendants were eleven manufacturers of asbestos-containing insulation products, including Johns-Manville, Fibreboard, Eagle-Picher, and Owens Corning. The complaint alleged that although the defendants either knew or should have known that their products were harmful to human health, they failed to warn Tomplait of the danger. The "failure to warn" element of the case would remain the centerpiece of the tens of thousands of legal suits that were to be filed against the asbestos industry in the decades to come.

During the trial, doctors testified that Tomplait's disease was progressive and irreversible and that he would gradually suffocate, and there wasn't anything medically to be done to prevent it. Tomplait testified that when he coughed it felt as though he were being stuck by a thousand needles. (In reality, he vastly underestimated the number.) Some of the defendants had already been dropped from the complaint, and five more agreed to settle. Although the case against the sixth and final defendant, Fibreboard, was the weakest from the plaintiff's point of view, and the verdict was ultimately returned in favor of the defendant, Tomplait's attorney, Ward Stephenson, sensed that the asbestos manufacturers were vulnerable.

In October 1969, Stephenson, this time representing a workmate of Tomplait's, Clarence Borel, filed in federal district court in Beaumont for damages of $1 million against eleven asbestos-insulation manufacturers, including most of the same companies in the Tomplait case, plus Unarco, Combustion Engineering, and the Philip Carey Corporation. *Clarence Borel v. Fibreboard Paper Products Corporation et al.* would become the most famous asbestos litigation case in history. At the heart of the dispute was the "failure to warn" charge, plus the allegation that the companies had not removed the products from the marketplace when they were found to be dangerous.

Borel, who suffered from an advanced case of mesothelioma, died before his trial but was able to give a deposition from his bed shortly before his death on June 3, 1970. The trial began in September 1971, after Unarco, Eagle-Picher, Owens Corning, and Standard Asbestos had settled out of court. Most of the critical testimony and strategy involved the witnesses testifying for Johns-Manville. It was during the Borel trial that the asbestos industry first employed a tactic that proved relatively effective for fifteen years, until plaintiff attorneys made a sensational find in a musty old closet that tore the strategy apart and caused a well-founded panic among the industry.

The tactic was first used during a telling exchange between Johns-Manville's accident-prevention manager, Clifford Scheckler, and Stephenson. In a daylong session, Scheckler stuck to his testimony that the first time he had ever heard that asbestos was dangerous to human health was during the presentation of Dr. Selikoff's findings at the 1964 New York Academy of Sciences conference. Despite hours of grilling by Stephenson, Scheckler refused to budge from his statements. This tactic was to become known as the "state of the art" defense. Scores of defense witness from that time forward followed Scheckler's lead and testified that they did not know of the dangers of asbestos before Selikoff's research. The implications, of course, were that they therefore could not be held liable for the illness of any worker exposed before 1964.

Scheckler, whose wife would later die of mesothelioma, told the jury that it had not occurred to the management at Johns-

Manville that people who did not work at fixed positions during their shift could suffer pulmonary disease.

Stephenson, a tough, gritty fighter, countered by introducing nearly ninety scientific and medical articles published before 1940—and readily available to the company's medical directors— that outlined, in detail, the dangers of asbestos. He also rebutted the defense's argument that the workers did not use the available safety equipment, such as respirators, by producing Borel's deposition. In it, Borel stated that although he sometimes put Mentholatum in his nostrils and wore a handkerchief around his face to keep out the heavy dust, he and the other workers did not believe— nor were they ever told by management—that the asbestos dust was dangerous.

In a landmark decision, Stephenson won the case, but it was quickly appealed to the 5th Circuit Court. Although few people knew it, Stephenson was suffering from cancer during the trial, and as the appeal ground its way through the legal process, the plaintiff attorney's health deteriorated. He argued the case in November 1972 and then waited anxiously for nearly a year before the decision was handed down. In September 1973, a week before Stephenson slipped into a coma and died, the court ruled in his client's favor. Judge John Wisdom wrote that product manufacturers have a responsibility to warn of "foreseeable dangers" associated with their products. "This duty to warn extends to all users and consumers, including the common worker in the shop or in the field," the judge wrote. "Here there was a duty to speak, but the defendants remained silent. The district court's judgment does no more than hold the defendants liable for the foreseeable consequences of their own inaction. . . . An insulation worker, no less than any other product user, has a right to decide whether to expose himself to the risk."

The court upheld the award of $79,436 to the plaintiff. The

Borel trial marked the first case ever won in the United States by an asbestos victim.

Despite the victory in the Borel case, however, plaintiff attorneys found that the industry's "state of the art" defense often prevailed over their own "failure to warn" arguments. Even in cases where the plaintiffs triumphed, they were usually awarded relatively small amounts of money, and judges usually discouraged the awarding of punitive damages.

That all changed one spring day in 1977, when Karl Asch, a plaintiff's attorney from Springfield, New Jersey, made one of the strangest and most important discoveries in the history of American jurisprudence. While representing former employees from Raybestos-Manhattan's Passaic plant, Asch had come across a section in the company's 1974 annual report that strengthened his suspicion that the asbestos industry had long been guilty of a cover-up. As early as 1930, Raybestos-Manhattan had commissioned the Metropolitan Life Insurance Company to survey all its factories and to make recommendations for the elimination of conditions that might present health hazards. Long-range research programs on the health effects of asbestos were then funded by the industry. The report spurred Asch to subpoena the CEO of Raybestos-Manhattan, William Simpson, the son of the company founder, Sumner Simpson. It was during that deposition that Asch was to make the greatest discovery of all.

During questioning, Simpson admitted that his father had retained Saranac Laboratories to do animal studies involving the harmful effects of asbestos. When Asch asked where the records of the studies were kept, he was startled to hear that those records, along with a carton of Sumner Simpson's personal documents, were stored in Simpson's Bridgeport, Connecticut, office. They had remained secure in a locked closet there for nearly thirty years. When

Asch obtained copies of the files during the discovery phase of the trial, he was shocked. There were thousands of documents, including a complete record of the communications between the Browns at Johns-Manville and Sumner Simpson. Apparently Simpson had saved nearly every scrap of correspondence during his time as CEO, and his son, according to Asch, "respected his father deeply and wouldn't have dreamed of destroying any of his records." The documents in the old box in the musty closet became known as the Sumner Simpson Papers, and they blew apart the asbestos industry's "state of the art" defense. They were later nicknamed "The Asbestos Pentagon Papers" by plaintiff lawyers. "Whatever you call them," Asch told author Brodeur, "they were collectively a smoking gun."

The documents revealed in clear detail the fraud and conspiracy the two companies, and the asbestos industry as a whole, had perpetuated since the 1930s. The efforts to censor the trade media were exposed, as well as the cover-up of the various medical tests done that showed widespread asbestos-related diseases among the workers.

Federal judge Harold Ackerman of New Jersey, in *Anna Billetz et al. v. Johns-Manville* (Civ. No. 80-2976), later found that the study by Dr. Lanza at the Metropolitan Life Insurance Company was altered "apparently in accordance with the asbestos industry's wishes." The judge said one of the "most glaring alterations" was the deletion of the conclusion that "it is possible for uncomplicated asbestosis to result fatally."

In total, the Sumner Simpson letters were so damaging to the asbestos industry that, according to Barry Castleman, South Carolina circuit judge James Price granted a new trial in one asbestos damage suit already won by the defendants. Judge Price stated: "The correspondence very arguably shows a pattern of denial and disease and attempts at suppression of information which is highly probative."

The damage done to the defendants from these documents was

monumental. First, it destroyed the "state of the art" defense put forth by Scheckler and dozens of other top asbestos industry officials that they didn't know of the asbestos dangers until the 1964 Selikoff studies. Second, it further exposed the industry's culpability and opened the floodgates to a tidal wave of litigation.

An estimated six hundred thousand lawsuits have been filed against the asbestos industry since that time. Plaintiff lawyers and their investigators continue to reveal the industry's efforts to hide the dangers of asbestos from the American people. The Florida Supreme Court in 1999 summed up the strategies of Owens Corning in a way that applied to the entire industry. "It would be difficult to envision a more egregious set of circumstances . . . a blatant disregard for human safety involving large numbers of people put at life-threatening risk." *(Opinion No. 92,963, August 26, 1999.)*

Among the Sumner Simpson letters was a letter from Simpson to an executive at the Thermoid Rubber Company discussing the asbestos studies being done at Saranac Labs. Simpson and J-M president Lewis Brown were concerned about possible negative publicity from the tests. In the letter, Simpson explained that he and Brown had hatched a plan to have asbestos manufacturers take over the study so they could determine whether to publish the findings. Simpson said he thought it was a good idea to "distribute the information among the medical fraternity, providing it is of the right type and would not injure our companies."

Correspondence outlining the successful attempts by Brown and Simpson to censor both the studies and the publication of asbestos information in trade magazines was included, as were their letters to Saranac Labs, including one that stated: "It is our further understanding that the result obtained will be considered the property of those who are advancing the required funds, who will determine, whether, to what extent, and in what manner they shall be made public."

The confidentiality agreement between J-M and the U.S. Public Health Service, stating that none of the X rays of J-M workers taken by the Health Service could be revealed to those workers—lest they fall into the hands of "shyster lawyers"—was also there.

The discovery by plaintiff attorneys also revealed that the suppression of health documents outlining the hazards of asbestos was a routine strategy for the asbestos industry, J-M in particular. Even the application of warning labels, which J-M corporate medical director Dr. Kenneth Smith recommended in 1952, was resisted by the company. Dr. Smith later testified that the company decision on including warning labels was made in a similar fashion industry-wide. Smith stated:

> The reason why the caution labels were not implemented immediately, it was a business decision as far as I could understand. Here was a recommendation, the corporation is in business to make, to provide jobs for people and make money for stockholders and they had to take into consideration the effects of everything they did and if the application of a caution label identifying a product as hazardous would cut into sales, there would be serious financial implications. And the powers of be [sic] had to make some effort to judge the necessity of the label versus the consequences of placing the label on the product. (K. W. Smith deposition in Louisville Trust Co. v. Johns-Manville Corp. Jefferson Circuit Court, Common Pleas Br. 7th Div. of Kentucky, Case No 174-922, April 21, 1976.)

Additional revelations of the industry's fatal deception, reprinted with permission and presented below, are to be found in Asbestos: Medical and Legal Aspects by Barry Castleman (Aspen Law

and Business, 1996). These cases show how for a span of seven
decades an entire industry willfully disregarded the health of American workers and consumers.

When Eagle-Picher Industries began making an asbestos-
containing cement called Super 66 in 1938, the dangers of asbestos
were already well known to the company. A report to the company
by the U.S. Bureau of Mines in 1932 stated that lung fibrosis was
found among asbestos workers in the company's plant in Joplin,
Missouri. "It is now known that asbestos dust is one of the most
dangerous dusts to which man is exposed," the report stated. Despite that early warning and all the subsequent medical studies that
showed asbestos to be deadly, the company refused to acknowledge
the problem. In a May 22, 1968, letter to the Shell Oil Company,
E-P executives stated: "The above Eagle-Picher products [Super 66
and another asbestos-containing cement called One-Cote] do not
contain toxic ingredients. Therefore, no antidotes are needed." The
asbestos remained in the cements for nearly thirty years, in spite
of the fact that asbestos was never a critical component in the
product, according to retired company engineer Herman Lee
Huelster. Huelster testified that the company used asbestos as a
"sales gimmick." He also testified that the requirement for asbestos
in some naval specifications for insulating cements was not the
result of technical need but rather the "clout" of the asbestos
industry.

In 1947, a study titled "A Report of Preliminary Dust Investigation for the Asbestos Textile Institute" stated that 20 percent of the
workers in two of five J-M plants tested had asbestosis. The report
indicated that findings were similar industry-wide.

In November 1948, A. J. Vorwald of Saranac Laboratories
wrote a letter to W. E. Bowes, the director of research for Owens-
Illinois, regarding asbestos tests done there on guinea pigs. It stated,
in part: "In all animals sacrificed after more than thirty months of

exposure to Kaylo dust, unmistakable evidence of asbestosis has developed, showing that Kaylo on inhalation is capable of producing asbestosis and must be regarded as a potentially-hazardous material." The letter ends by stating: "I realize that our findings regarding Kaylo are less favorable than anticipated. However, since Kaylo is capable of producing asbestosis, it is better to discover it now in animals rather than later in industrial workers. Thus the company, being forewarned, will be in a better position to institute adequate control measures for safeguarding exposed employees and protecting its own interests."

Despite this specific medical finding, on December 9, 1952, an intracompany memo circulated that contained a draft of a proposed pamphlet on Kaylo intended for public use. It stated: "There is no danger of developing asbestosis with normal handling of Kaylo products." It concluded, "Experience in the factories and field and research findings have proven that normal handling of Kaylo products is safe from a health standpoint."

An internal company memo in 1963 admitted that the asbestos in Kaylo "when breathed into the lungs causes asbestosis which often leads to lung cancer." The following year, Owens-Corning Fiberglas circulated internal memos stating that the company needed to find a way of preventing Dr. Selikoff from creating problems and affecting sales. Tens of thousands of lawsuits were filed against Owens Corning (Owens-Illinois) in the 1980s and 1990s in large part because the company concealed early knowledge that Kaylo was a dangerous product.

A medical consultant for Southern Textile of Charlotte, North Carolina, which manufactured a number of asbestos products, provided this startling finding in a trade journal in 1955: "The pessimism of the past is being replaced by the realization that a diagnosis of silicosis or asbestosis is compatible with good health and a feeling of well-being."

Philip Carey Manufacturing of Cincinnati, which supplied asbestos and asbestos products to Americans since 1880, became concerned over potential legal problems stemming from the asbestos in its products and in the early 1960s hired Dr. Thomas Mancuso to study the health hazards to the company's workers and customers. In 1964, Dr. Mancuso wrote a report to the company's legal department that contained the following:

> *There is an irrefutable association between asbestos and cancer. This association has been established for cancer of the lung and for mesothelioma. There is suggestive evidence . . . for cancer of the stomach, colon and rectum, also. There is substantial evidence that cancer and mesothelioma have developed in environmentally exposed groups, i.e., due to air pollution for groups living near asbestos plants and mines.* [Had this information been passed on to W. R. Grace—and then acted upon in a moral and responsible manner—hundreds and perhaps thousands of lives could have been saved in Libby, Montana, and elsewhere.] *Evidence has been established for cancer developing among members of the household. Mesotheliomas have developed among wives, laundering the work clothes of asbestos workers. Substantial evidence has been presented that slight and intermittent exposures may be sufficient to produce lung cancer and mesothelioma. There should be no delusion that the problem will disappear or that the consumer or working population will not become aware of the problem and the compensation and legal liability involved.*

Soon after this letter was received, Philip Carey fired Dr. Mancuso.

Union Carbide operated chrysotile asbestos mines in California from 1963 through 1985. The asbestos was used in drywall patching compounds, plastics, and paints. A 1966 study on the dangers of asbestos in Union Carbide's United Kingdom operations was found years later in a library in Montreal with an index card on it that read, "Confidential—not circulated." In a part of the report entitled "Moral Issues" the author wrote: "On the basis of present evidence we are not entitled under any circumstances to state that our material is not a health hazard. What is more, if it is believed that a potential customer would use our material 'dangerously,' and that he is unaware of the toxicity question, then it must surely be our duty to caution him and point out means whereby he can hold the asbestos air float concentration to a minimum." In fact, Union Carbide asbestos containers did not bear warning labels until 1971, and in 1977, the company led a fight against the proposed ban on the use of asbestos in drywall spackling and joint compounds.

In a particularly frightening piece of correspondence on September 12, 1966, the director of purchasing for Allied Signal (Bendix) wrote to J-M executives: "My answer to the problem is: If you have enjoyed a good life while working with asbestos products, why not die from it? There's got to be some cause."

Also in 1966, J-M executive M. Snowcroft wrote the following to Bath Iron Works: "We feel that the recent unfavorable publicity over the use of asbestos fibers in many different kinds of industries has been a gross exaggeration of the problems. There is no data available to either prove or disprove the dangers of working closely with asbestos."

Bath Iron Works executives must have wondered what was going on because on August 8, 1966, Owens-Corning Fiberglas executives wrote to the company citing Dr. Selikoff's belief that only one asbestos fiber can cause cancer and suggested that the company begin to label Kaylo products, much as J-M labeled theirs beginning in 1964. In 1970, warning labels were finally placed on packages of

Kaylo, acknowledging explicitly that the dust could be harmful. Yet in 1972, OCF bought 145 tons of amosite asbestos.

"Unibestos contains amosite asbestos which has thus far not been incriminated as a producer of asbestosis." This total fabrication was contained in a 1966 letter from the medical director of the Pittsburgh Corning Corporation to the managers of Bath Iron Works. The truth is that the amosite used in the insulation at the plant in Tyler, Texas, run by Pittsburgh Corning was highly toxic. The story of the Tyler plant is one of mind-boggling deception and death. In 1962, Unarco sold the plant to Pittsburgh Corning. Ongoing surveys by U.S. occupational health and safety inspectors showed that conditions in the plant were unhealthy for workers, but once again the government inspectors were working under a confidentiality agreement with the company, and none of the workers were notified. A decade went by, and several different government studies continued to indicate that the health hazards inside the plant were severe. Finally, when more than 40 percent of the men with more than ten years of employment at the mine were found to have asbestosis, the government stepped in and fined the company—$210. In 1972, the plant in Tyler was shut down and found to be so contaminated with asbestos fibers that the entire facility was simply buried. So too were more than an estimated one-third of the 895 workers at the plant, fatalities of the dust that was "not a producer of asbestosis." For its part, Unarco had operated a similar plant in Paterson, New Jersey, which was closed in 1954. Dr. Selikoff tracked seventeen of the men who had worked at the Paterson plant, and by 1974, all but two had died of asbestos-related diseases. Despite the numerous reports of health hazards at the Paterson plant, when Unarco opened the Tyler plant, it was not criticized or monitored by the government; indeed, according to Brodeur, it was rewarded with huge U.S. Navy contracts to provide amosite-asbestos pipe coverings for nuclear submarines.

From 1975 through 1977, a series of internal J-M memos acknowledged the danger of "high dust levels" in brake repair and expressed the need to assure that warnings reached the repair shops nationwide. Castleman wrote: "The second memo, marked 'CONFIDENTIAL,' noted that 'exposure to excessive levels [of asbestos] for a few months or even a few weeks can result in the appearance of disease many years later.' This memo also stressed the importance of preventing workers from taking dust home on their clothes. The last memo advised against telling customers that asbestos products could be used safely. 'We cannot use the word safe simply because we do not know what a safe level of exposure is.'"

In 1976, after the EPA banned asbestos-containing molded insulation, Keene offered another company a discount on its remaining asbestos-containing products to be exported "outside the continental U.S." Samples of Keene products at the Amerada Hess oil refinery on the island of Saint Croix, labeled "asbestos-free," were found in 1982 to contain large amounts of amosite asbestos.

The corporate guilt and the onslaught of legal suits that followed weren't restricted to American companies. In England, Turner & Newall, once the "asbestos giant" of the world, was hammered with lawsuits as the same revelations about concealment of danger and failure to warn were being revealed by plaintiff attorneys.

The tide against the asbestos industry in England turned in July 1982, when a powerful documentary was aired on British television. *Alice—A Fight for Life* was a moving two-hour tale of Alice Jefferson, a forty-seven-year-old Yorkshire mother who had worked for only a few months in the Hebden Bridge asbestos plant, one of the dustiest and most dangerous in England. Jefferson, who died a brave but excruciatingly painful death of mesothelioma, became a symbol of the gross negligence of the industry. Wrote Geoffrey Tweedale, in *Magic Mineral to Killer Dust: Turner & Newall and the Asbestos Hazard* (Oxford University Press, 2000):

> *Even after nearly thirty years the documentary has not lost its power to shock. Its main subject was death; unpleasant enough in any circumstances, but particularly so when it involved the dreadful physical misery of asbestos cancer victims. Besides Alice's final days, which were followed to their inevitable end in the cemetery, viewers were confronted by the sight of children and young adults cut down by mesothelioma; they saw the Cape manager (himself an asbestosis sufferer), who always kept a black tie in his desk for funerals; . . . they saw the dissembling of doctors; the tightfistedness of the government and the denials of the asbestos companies.*

The documentary sent asbestos sales reeling and soon T&N, the once seemingly invincible asbestos giant, was on the financial ropes. By the end of 1982, the Bank of England had to organize a rescue to keep T&N from bankruptcy. By the 1990s, asbestos claims against the company—which Tweedale characterized as "once paid *ex gratia* from loose change at the head office"—were skyrocketing into the millions of pounds.

One of the worst examples of deliberate corporate contamination, however, happened halfway across the world in a mining town in the western Australian outback where events eerily foreshadowed what was to happen in Libby. From the 1940s until 1966, when the mine closed, the town of Wittenoom was polluted with asbestos fibers, exposing tens of thousands of men, women, and children.

The huge deposit of blue crocidolite asbestos in the Wittenoom Gorge in the Pilbara region was mined by the Australian Blue Asbestos Company, a subsidiary of the Colonial Sugar Refinery (CSR), one of Australia's largest corporations. CSR ran a deadly operation, even when judged by asbestos industry standards. The dust inside the underground mine was reported to be so thick that workers sometimes hurt themselves when they ran into equipment or frameworks they couldn't see. Residents recalled a constant opaque cloud from the mine hanging over the town, where some twenty thousand lived when the mine was operational. It shut down in 1966, not because of gross violations of human occupational safety laws, but because of declining economic conditions. During the nearly three decades of operation, the mine produced more than 150,000 tons of some of the world's deadliest asbestos.

In the late 1940s, the mine was visited by managers from America's Johns-Manville plant in New Jersey. Whether this was a coincidence, a short time later CSR asked the Australian Immigration Department to help provide immigrant workers for the mine. J-M, of course, had successfully used immigrant workers in Manville and in other U.S. plants. Italian, Yugoslav, Dutch, German, Greek, Hungarian, Polish, and Spaniard immigrants—nearly all penniless and desperately seeking jobs—were sent to Wittenoom on two-year employment bonds.

The multiple exposure pathways ultimately encountered by the Wittenoom residents are similar to those that poisoned residents of Libby. Poor ventilation in the mining shed exposed workers to clouds of asbestos dust every hour they were on the job. The town was saturated with mine tailings and asbestos. As in Libby, the children of Wittenoom learned to write their names in the asbestos dust on the sidewalks of the town.

The Australian government was as impotent as the Montana regulatory agencies when it came to enforcement measures. Ben Hills, an investigative reporter whose book *Blue Murder* (Sun Books,

1989) chronicled the terrible events of the Wittenoom story, stated that the government did little to clean up or close the mine. Like its American counterparts, it did nothing "during the life of the mine or the death of its workers" to make CSR accountable. It was left to the dying families to seek justice through the court systems.

Val Doyle, a forty-nine-year-old woman who lived in Wittenoom, told Hills that the poisoning of the town had been deliberate and profitable. Her words could well be etched in granite on a monument on Mineral Avenue in Libby, for everyone in that town has said or heard them a thousand times. "They knew what was going on," she said. "The doctors knew. The company knew. The only people they never told was us . . . and now we are dying. I call it criminal."

Doyle died a few weeks after she made that statement. She was the sixth member of her family to die from asbestos poisoning at Wittenoom.

No safety measures were ever recorded by the company, even though the workers' unions often bitterly complained to the government. The inspectors would often respond to the complaints by flying in to Wittenoom, the only timely way to reach the town. The problem was, the only airline available to the area was run by the mining company. The mine managers were informed as soon as the inspectors made their reservations. By the time they arrived, the mine was cleaned and wetted down.

Nearly two thousand former Wittenoom residents have already died from asbestos-related diseases, and the number is expected to continue to rise. Asbestos fibers were found even in the lungs of newborn babies, so the Wittenoom legacy is assured victims into the next generation. After the mine closed, the town was found to be so saturated with asbestos fibers that 220 buildings had to be demolished by workers in HazMat suits. These included

the hospital, hotel, bank, cinemas, racetrack, and a number of residences.

Today, Wittenoom is a boarded-up ghost town and a macabre
tourist attraction. A few dozen residents still live there and offer
motel and restaurant services for a surprising number of curious
visitors who travel to see the site of Australia's worst industrial disaster, even though airborne asbestos in the area remains a potential
problem.

In the United States, companies, many of which manufactured no
asbestos-containing materials themselves but which bought or
merged with companies that did, complain bitterly about the hundreds of thousands of lawsuits still being filed against them by victims and alleged victims. The Rand Corporation estimates that as
many as 1.5 million lawsuits may ultimately be filed. Lost in the current uproar over the number of lawsuits is the key reason for their
existence: the obvious and horrific guilt of most of the asbestos
companies. The court findings in some of the cases already decided
for the plaintiffs are as damning as one might expect.

U.S. DISTRICT COURT FOR NEW JERSEY: "The Saranac
studies, and the possible link of asbestos to cancer, were discussed
at proceedings of the National Cancer Institute in January of 1944,
but the ultimate report was published only in 1951. The published
report omitted references to human asbestosis and cancer, as well
as the finding that there was no safe level of exposure to asbestos.
Moreover, through their lobbying activities, members of the asbestos industry assured the public that asbestos products in their
buildings posed no health hazard. Yet a memorandum from W. R.
Grace's manager of fireproofing products to senior management

stated that 'we have an ethical obligation to get asbestos out.'"
(Prudential Ins. Co. v. U.S. Gypsum, 828 F. Supp. 287 [D.N.J. 1993].)

APPELLATE COURT OF ILLINOIS: "The evidence showed that defendant was aware of the hazards of asbestos, chose not to disclose the information, and failed to place warning labels on the product at the time it knew of the hazards of the product. . . . It is also evident that defendant continued to hesitate to place warning labels on the products as late as 1970, even after they became aware of the possibility of lawsuits. This conduct clearly amounts to an utter indifference to, or conscious disregard for the safety of others." *(Kochan v. Owens-Corning Fiberglas Corp., 610 N.E. 2d 683, 1993.)*

SUPREME COURT OF NEW JERSEY: "It is indeed appalling to us that Johns-Manville had so much information on the hazards to asbestos workers as early as the 1930's and that it not only failed to use that information to protect these workers but, more egregiously, that it also attempted to withhold this information from the public." *(Fischer v. Johns-Manville, 512 A. 2nd 466 [N.J. 1986].)*

COURT OF APPEALS OF FLORIDA: "The evidence in this case . . . is sufficient to establish that Johns-Manville had knowledge, at least from the decade of the 1930's, that prolonged exposure to asbestos dust and fibers would cause the chronic lung disease commonly known as asbestosis. In the early 1900's, it was known that asbestos could cause lung disease, a report thereof having been published in 1907. . . . Johns-Manville had a policy of not telling employees about the results of X-rays that showed that they were suffering from asbestosis, so they 'can live and work in peace and the company can benefit by their many years of experience.'" *(Janssens v. Johns-Manville, 463, So. 2nd 242: Florida 1984.)*

FLORIDA APPELLATE COURT: "There is voluminous evidence that the asbestos industry has known for decades of the dangers involved in the use of asbestos products." *(Copeland v. Celotex, 447 S. 2nd 908: Florida App. 1984.)*

U.S. DISTRICT COURT FOR EASTERN DISTRICT OF TEXAS: "The asbestos industry, composed of many manufacturers, has introduced hundreds of products into the stream of commerce which are, either by design or failure to warn, unreasonably dangerous for their intended use." *(Migues v. Nicolet Industries, 493 F. Supp. 61: E.D. Tex. 1980.)*

U.S. DISTRICT COURT FOR EASTERN DISTRICT OF VIRGINIA: "The plaintiff introduced evidence tending to establish that the defendant manufacturers either were, or should have been, fully aware of the many articles and studies on asbestosis. The evidence also indicated, however, that during [the plaintiff's] working career no manufacturer ever warned contractors or insulation workers, including [the plaintiff], of the dangers associated with inhaling asbestos dust." *(Borel v. Fibreboard Paper Products, 493 F. 2d 1076: 5th Cir. 1973.)*

As the mountain of evidence against the asbestos industry grew, juries became increasingly outraged at the industry's complete disregard for their workers and their customers. In many cases, proving the asbestos companies' absolute guilt was not difficult for plaintiff lawyers. Much of the time the game was over for the defense lawyers before it began. Juries throughout the country were furious at what many felt was the criminal behavior of the executives of the asbestos companies.

Brodeur noted that in 1980, John McKinney, Johns-Manville's chairman and CEO, based his argument regarding J-M's innocence on the fact that no jury had ever awarded punitive damages against the company. He neglected to add that judges had routinely discouraged punitive damage awards. McKinney was forced to eat his words a year later when a federal-court jury awarded a claimant $450,000 dollars in punitive damages in a case against Johns-Manville and Celotex. By the mid-1980s, as the entire story of the J-M cover-up unfolded, million-dollar awards against the company were not uncommon.

Even today, asbestos apologists like to say that the true cost of the hundreds of thousands of lawsuits being filed lies within the legal proceedings themselves, not with any fear of losing in court. But the truth is, juries were often stunned at the litany of malfeasance perpetrated by the asbestos companies and have delivered scores of huge plaintiff awards especially to mesothelioma victims, who usually face hundreds of thousands of dollars in medical debts.

A sampling of some of the most recent jury awards include:

- A $5.4 million verdict for a Texas construction worker with mesothelioma, 2001.
- $4.9 million to a Minnesota laborer with mesothelioma, 2001.
- $4.5 million to a Texas laborer with mesothelioma, 2001.
- $6.3 million to a California woman with mesothelioma who was exposed in her home, 2001.
- $2.3 million to a California woman with asbestosis, 2001.
- $6 million to a Louisiana pipe fitter with mesothelioma, 2000.

- $5.4 million to a Texas steelworker with mesothelioma, 2000.
- $5 million to a Texas woman with mesothelioma exposed through her father's trade, 2000.
- $4.6 million to a U.S. Navy seaman with mesothelioma, 2000.
- $3.7 to a California carpenter with mesothelioma, 2000.
- $3.77 million to a Texas pipe fitter with mesothelioma, 2000.
- $3.6 million to a Kansas pipe fitter with mesothelioma, 2000.
- $2.8 million to a U.S. Navy storekeeper from Georgia with mesothelioma, 2000.

The message that juries across the country have sent to asbestos companies is clear and unmistakable. At the same time, for every plaintiff's verdict there are scores of asbestos victims who, because of the arcane and archaic system of workers' compensation laws in some states or because their illness was misdiagnosed by physicians, never received a penny for the intense physical and mental anguish they suffered.

Vicki Kelley of Brunswick, Maine, knows of the true costs involved in losing a loved one to asbestos. When her father, William Wallace, died of mesothelioma on November 18, 1998, the local newspaper called him "The Mayor of Main Street." Nearly everyone in Brunswick knew "Wally," as he preferred to be called. He was a major part of the tapestry of the town. He was the founder of the town's recreation department and helped build the town library. He was the president of the PTA, a Little League umpire, and a soft touch for a couple of bucks for an ice-cream cone. He sang off-tune every Sunday at the Methodist church, and the bookstore where he had worked for so long closed for good the day after he died.

"My dad loved this town and I believe the town loved him,"

said Vicki. "He wasn't ready to die. He had so many things left that he wanted to do. He wanted to help his grandchildren grow up."

Wally spent a year, as a young man, working for Bath Iron Works, one of the largest shipbuilding companies in the country, as an electrician's helper. He crawled through the small, narrow spaces on some of the old shipbuilding plants, pulling out the old asbestos insulation so the electrician could run his wires. The insulation often fell apart in his hands, sending small clouds of dust up around him. He was reassured that the dust wouldn't hurt him.

After his brief stint with Bath Iron Works, Wally went to work managing a local bookstore, where he spent his career. "He had to quit high school in the ninth grade so he could support his mother," recalled Vicki. "But he had always loved books, and he never stopped learning. He even took a course in new math as we were growing up, so he could help us out with our homework. I know it wasn't easy for him, but he did it for us."

Everything seemed fine when Wally retired, although he had chronic lung problems that his doctor originally diagnosed as asthma. His constant coughing and frequent pain didn't prevent him from attending all his grandchildren's sporting events. His lung problems persisted, however, and Wally finally saw a specialist in July 1998. Vicki drove him to the medical appointment, and she remembers the numbing words of the doctor. "Mr. Wallace," the doctor said, "you have a massive and inoperative tumor in your chest." Wally had a disease neither he nor Vicki had ever heard of before, one that the doctor explained was irreversible and quick acting. Wally was advised to put his affairs in order.

That night, after Vicki took her father home, she sat in her bedroom too stunned to cry. As the days went by she found some solace in writing down her thoughts. Her first words were: "My father is dying. What a strange sentence that is. He has mesothelioma . . . isn't that a pretty name? When you say it aloud it sounds so lovely . . . it flows beautifully off the tongue. And it will kill him in an ugly way. I am not ready."

The disease hit Wally hard. He had his lungs drained so regularly that he finally underwent a painful operation to "seal" them in an attempt to keep them from filling with liquid. The huge tumor in the pleura lining grew rapidly, pushing and restricting and finally crushing his lung. Vicki took an extended leave of absence from her job to be with her father. She drove him through the neighborhood streets where he used to walk every day. He never complained, never asked "Why me?" and never showed that he was in constant pain.

"He didn't hate and he wasn't angry at those of us who got to live," said Vicki. "It helped that the whole town was there for him. They threw parties in his honor, and people came by to see him all the time. Just before he died we took him to my ten-year-old son's football game. My son played quarterback, and the coach knew Dad didn't have much time so he made sure my son got in some big plays. Dad appreciated the attention, but he wasn't ready to die."

Near the end, Wally's health failed so badly that he went into the hospital. Vicki remembers walking through the waiting room. "It was full of people whose relatives had mesothelioma," she said. "The incredible grief that disease causes is more than I can think about even now. It is a death sentence for the entire family."

Although it has been four years since her father died, Vicki still has not been able to accept his death. The more she learns about how much the asbestos companies knew and didn't tell their workers, the more difficult it becomes.

"All they would have had to do is provide him with the proper protective equipment, and he would still be alive and with us today," she said. "My level of anger is pretty extreme. All those legal cases prove that they knew that asbestos causes lung cancer. They knew it. How hard would it have been to have given my dad and the rest of the workers respirators and protective clothing? How hard? How dare they put people's lives in jeopardy, and then go home every night to their cozy houses and their happy little families and live their lives out. They killed thousands of people and nothing is being done about it, except they lose some court cases and have to pay some money. Is that money worth my father's life? He and my mother were married for fifty-four years. Now she doesn't know what to do. She just sits at home and waits. They played God with people's lives."

11

THE EPA
LANDS IN LIBBY

*"One of the reasons asbestos companies have gotten away
with what they have for so many years is the victims are
often old men. We tolerate them dying in occupational positions all the time. Old men die pretty quietly. But, if you
watch how they die from asbestos, it's hard, really hard."*

—Paul Peronard

A year after her mother's death in Libby, Gayla Benefield had still
not gotten over her grief and anger. Despite the fact she had
been the first person in Libby to successfully sue W. R. Grace, she felt
as though she had failed. Her promise had not been kept. She hadn't
stopped or exposed Grace. They had skated by with a minimal
payout. It was a wound that wouldn't heal.

In the early fall of 1999, the trees were already turning spectacular colors in the Cabinet Mountains. The mornings were chilly,
and Benefield grasped a hot mug of coffee as she read the local
paper. She glanced in anger at a story outlining how Grace was
nearing the end of the cleanup of the mine, which it had abandoned
in 1990, years after overwhelming evidence had surfaced that the

vermiculite was contaminated with asbestos. Vermiculite had been excavated as late as 1987.

But in the fall of 1999, the mine was quiet. Rope swings still hung from the old buildings at the abandoned popping plant at the north edge of town, and kids still played there on occasion, among the abandoned piles of vermiculite. A commercial nursery was now operating on the site of the old screening plant on the banks of the Kootenai, where Bob Wilkins once worked.

As Benefield sipped her coffee and read on, a familiar number caught her eye. Grace had posted a cleanup bond years before and was filing to recover the unused portion. It came to $67,000—the same amount she had received in the lawsuit over her mother's death! The odd coincidence jolted her upright. A thought raced through her mind: If Grace had tried to cover up the truth about what it did to the workers on the mountain, why would it tell the truth about the cleanup? She grabbed her car keys and did something she hadn't done for thirty years—she drove to the mine. When she got there, what she saw off Rainy Creek Road didn't surprise her. The area didn't look reclaimed at all. Water was running through the highly contaminated tailings into Rainy Creek and into the river. The area was a mess, with exposed tailings just waiting for the slightest wind to release their deadly fibers into the air.

Benefield drove quickly home, her mind a mix of anger and excitement. Despite what she knew about Grace, she was still amazed at the company's arrogance. It was literally thumbing its nose at the Montana state inspectors. She immediately dialed the numbers for the state regulatory agencies, which she had come to know so well. When she finally got through, no one seemed interested. They told her to file an official complaint, which she did. She received a bureaucratic stiff arm for three weeks that only made her madder. "I cussed them out and raised hell," she said later. "Somebody had to do something."

Finally, on September 13, 1999, state officials caved in to her relentless phone calls and went to the mine and found it exactly as Benefield had described. Seizing the opportunity, Benefield contacted the press. This time, she hit pay dirt.

When the phone rang in their Denver home, Tracy Peronard moved past her husband, who was sprawled on the living room floor, to answer it. Paul had fallen while rock climbing the day before and was icing a sore back, his feet up on a chair. Tracy talked for a moment, and then Paul watched as her face fell. He could tell from the conversation that it was his boss at the EPA, Steve Hawthorne. Hawthorne told Tracy that he was going to e-mail Paul a series of recent newspaper articles about people getting sick from asbestos poisoning in a small town in Montana. Tracy had never heard of Libby. Her mind was on the Thanksgiving holiday, which was just days away. She had invited her entire family to the house for dinner and wanted Paul to be there. "He will be able to take care of things and be back by Thanksgiving, won't he?" she asked. Hawthorne thought that was a good possibility.

The next day, as Paul flew into Kalispell, about a ninety-minute drive east of Libby, he was perplexed. Lynette Hintze of the *Daily Inter Lake* and Andrew Schneider of the *Seattle Post-Intelligencer* had written articles indicating that something was terribly wrong in Libby—hundreds of people were dead or dying of asbestos exposure caused by the mine owned by W. R. Grace. To Benefield, who had contacted the media, the splashy stories had read like sweet redemption. To Peronard, they read like science fiction. In Peronard's fourteen years as an environmental hazards expert with the EPA, he had never heard of such fatality numbers, especially in a small town. The Seattle paper estimated that at least 192 people in Libby had died over the years due to asbestos-related diseases.

"Those numbers can't be right," Peronard thought, as his plane circled the thick forests surrounding Kalispell. "The reporters must have gotten carried away with some bad information."

A chemical engineer who had attended Georgia Tech, Peronard was a study of contrasts. He was thorough, analytical, and comfortable in the orderly world of numbers and scientific processes, yet he was an avid rock climber and HazMat expert, drawn to the energy and challenge of unpredictable and even dangerous environments. He had chosen a career within the bureaucracy, but he didn't fit the image. He shaved his once-long hair, wore showy earrings, and owned an impressive tattoo of Kokopelli, the Anasazi tribe's symbol of music, fertility, and good luck, on the underside of his muscled forearm. He wore hiking boots, sweatshirts, and blue jeans even to meetings, but his confidence and command was such that on a site, no one doubted that he was in charge. It was a unique combination of traits that made him a natural leader for the EPA's Region 8 Emergency Response Team.

Joining him in Libby were Chris Weis, a senior toxicologist and science coordinator out of the Denver EPA office, and Dr. Aubrey Miller, a physician and medical coordinator for the U.S. Public Health Service, Region 8. The Weis-Miller team was an intriguing one. They first worked together in 1998 on a project to help several Western states draw up bioterrorism plans. They found that they enjoyed working together and formed a bond of mutual respect. They had a lot in common. Both men were married, in their forties, and committed to their jobs. They found that by working together they were able to avoid a problem that had plagued many governmental environmental response teams. "Oftentimes the EPA guys don't know what the Health Service guys are doing, and vise versa," said Miller. "The lack of coordination can be serious in an emergency situation."

There was no model for their partnership, but they were able to convince their supervisors to allow them to continue to work together. (Their work became so highly regarded that Weis and Miller were chosen as lead members of the team that swept Senator Tom Daschle's office for anthrax two years later.)

Weis, an easygoing former medical school teacher, also had fourteen years with the EPA. He had been first on the scene at dozens of environmental disaster sites and was recognized as one of the top chemical "sleuths" in the country when it came to tracking down the source of poisonous pollutants. Miller, a talented environmental hazards expert with a medical degree, focused on the human health threats caused by the pollutants.

Weis and Miller were in Helena, Montana, finishing their work helping several Western states develop plans to deal with bioterrorism when the newspaper articles broke. Since they were already just a few hours away, they were told to head to Libby and link up with Peronard. Weis, who had worked with Peronard before, told Miller that he was a likable guy but was "kind of a cowboy" who sometimes threw away the bureaucratic book and did things his own way. Miller looked at Weis and grinned. He was looking forward to meeting this "cowboy."

By the time Weis and Miller arrived at the Super 8 Motel in Libby, it was dark and cold. They soon joined Peronard in his room that overlooked Highway 2, the only major east-west route through Libby. As they talked, the heater rattled trying to warm the air. Miller looked out into the freezing night and said that he hoped they would have the job wrapped up before the long Montana winter set in. Weis and Peronard nodded in agreement. What they couldn't have known was that Peronard's room was about to become an improbable "command center" for an improbable team about to come face-to-face with the largest and most lethal environmental disaster in American history.

The following day, November 23, 1999, the team met with city officials. They were assured that the newspaper articles had vastly overstated the problem. The Libby representatives were angry and felt that the articles had disparaged the city's reputation. On the surface, Libby looked fine. People were walking the streets and business seemed to be going on as usual. There was no evidence of strife or suffering anywhere. Mayor Anthony Berget summed up the town leaders' feelings in a quote that may well have echoed down throughout the asbestos mines and manufacturing plants for sixty years: If the asbestos contamination is that bad, the mayor said, "the state would have told us."

The EPA team had enough experience to know that in a town as remote as Libby, and in a state as antigovernment as Montana, environmental problems can sometimes go overlooked. A red flag went up when Peronard found that records showed Grace had already been fined $510,000 in 1994 for demolishing one of their contaminated buildings without notifying the EPA.

Later in the day, two men representing the Kootenai Development Company, which had purchased the abandoned vermiculite mine from Grace in hopes of logging it and eventually developing part of it into home sites, agreed to take the EPA team to the old mine.

"It was getting gloomy and cold by that time," recalled Miller. "Chris and I were riding in our rental car, and Paul was riding in a Blazer in front of us with the guys from KDC. We turned onto Rainy Creek Road, which was a dirt road then, and started winding our way up the mountain."

As they climbed higher, the wilderness suddenly cut away, and the men had a view down the mountainside. Ahead, the Blazer stopped and the KDC men got out. They were showing Peronard something, pointing over the ridge. Weis and Miller piled out, leaving the motor running to keep the car warm. As they slammed their doors shut, Miller got a funny feeling. He looked down and saw that his door was locked.

"Hey, Chris," he half-whispered, "my door locked." Weis looked back and, to his dismay, saw that his was locked also. "Shit!" he said, looking at Miller with horror on his face. The two highly trained field investigators stood still for a long moment before walking slowly over to where Peronard was pointing and talking with the other two men. Weis and Miller knew that government inspectors weren't exactly welcomed in that part of the country anyway, and now they had locked themselves out of their own running car in the middle of the freezing wilderness, and neither of them had on so much as a sweater.

"Uh, guys . . ." Weis began.

A spare key was driven out to them in less than an hour, but it was an inauspicious start for the crack EPA emergency response team.

During the next few days, Weis, Miller, and Peronard spread out across the town. Their initial findings surprised them. Weis and Peronard became concerned when they found bags of vermiculite still stacked at the popping plant, along with piles of stoner rock, the highly contaminated tailings left over when the vermiculite was heated. Some of the stoner rock was as much as 80 percent tremolite asbestos. The three men also talked to a number of residents, including Benefield. "She told us the story of her mother and father, and it just blew us away," said Miller.

By Thanksgiving, it was clear to the team that they were far from finished with their investigation. While the asbestos contamination was larger than they thought, they still weren't sure exactly what they had found in Libby. "It still seemed to us that most of the sick residents had been workers at the mine," said Peronard. "That was consistent with what we had seen in other areas. We were used to the idea that it was only the workers who were the ones exposed to high quantities of asbestos. We thought we might be up there another couple of months. We still weren't prepared for what was ahead."

After Thanksgiving, the team began tackling a number of challenges. Miller did a historical search for medical information and made a list of people to interview, most prominently Dr. Alan Whitehouse in Spokane.

Peronard and Weis began looking into the source and pathways of the asbestos pollution. The problem was that their experience was with industrial site pollution, not entire towns. Peronard was still skeptical of reports that so many nonworkers were sick in Libby. How could that be?

Samples at the mine revealed highly elevated levels of tremolite asbestos amphiboles. In fact, much of the mountain was tremolite, including boulders as big as city buses. In town, Peronard and Weis faced an immediate question. Should they test for asbestos fibers in the soil or the air?

"We considered the problem and determined that unequivocally, asbestos fibers make you sick if they are in the air and inhaled," said Weis. "So we put our monitors in the breathing zones. We felt we needed to first determine what the current exposure and risk was to the people of Libby."

Stationary monitors were set up around town at breathing levels, and some residents volunteered to wear smaller, portable monitors. "We wanted to reassure the people they weren't still at risk, but unfortunately, that isn't what we found," said Weis. "There were pockets of airborne fibers and some were in high concentrations."

Despite the high readings, Peronard felt that air sampling wasn't enough. He suspected there were other exposure pathways.

The team began questioning Libby residents, asking them to list all the ways in which they may have been exposed to vermiculite or the stoner rock. They needed to know how people might have actively contacted the fibers. That was the real clue as to the level of their exposure.

The answers they received surprised even Peronard. The vermiculite had been used in gardens, attics, walls, on driveways, and as fill around pipes and underground tanks—even as an ingredient in cookies. Many residents cited contact with vermiculite at the baseball fields and the popping plant. Peronard and Weis realized then that the contamination ranged far outside the mine.

By the end of December, the team had collected nearly seven hundred samples. This included air, soil, household dust, and insulation samples from private homes. Elevated tremolite fiber counts were found all over. Peronard found asbestos counts from trace levels to 15 percent in samples taken from the Libby baseball fields. Concentrations as low as 0.001 percent asbestos contamination in the soil have been reported to generate dangerous exposures, according to the EPA.

"We were growing more concerned with every finding, but the whole picture still hadn't yet emerged," Peronard said.

Meanwhile, Miller was receiving the results of several studies that he had ordered. He was driving back to the Super 8 Motel to read them when his cell phone rang. It was Bill Daniels, a colleague of Miller's who had discovered a paper discussing five cases of nonoccupational asbestos deaths. Daniels mentioned one in Minnesota where a man died at age forty-two from lung cancer and asbestosis. He said the victim's only known exposure to tremolite came from playing in a pile of stoner rock near a vermiculite processing plant in Minneapolis.

Miller almost drove his car off the road. "What!" he yelled, pulling over. "Tell me that again!" Miller knew the vermiculite had come from the Libby mine. He also knew there was a one-in-a-million chance that there would be a case study tying a case of asbestosis to Libby vermiculite. During the rest of his drive, Miller couldn't help but wonder: Was it just a coincidence, or was something going on here in Libby?

Back in his room, Miller began reading the background studies and was shocked at the amount of research that had already been done by the government and university researchers regarding the tremolite contamination of vermiculite. He couldn't help but wonder why somebody hadn't done something about it before now.

The following day, Miller and Michael Spence, the Montana state medical officer, made the four-hour drive to Spokane to interview Whitehouse. Miller was apprehensive about the meeting. Whitehouse had been outspoken in the local papers, giving numbers in the hundreds regarding the people he said he had treated for asbestos-related diseases in Libby. That sounded crazy to Miller, despite what Daniels had told him. Just what kind of doctor is this Whitehouse, he wondered. Hundreds of people with asbestos-related diseases in one small town? It didn't seem possible.

The interview was formal and somewhat tense. "Dr. Whitehouse clearly didn't want to be interrogated, and we were sizing him up," said Miller. "What we found was that he had the X rays, charts, and documentation that he said he did. He really knew his stuff. We came away impressed with him and suddenly very worried about what was happening in Libby."

During the early spring of 2000, the team was putting in sixteen-hour days. Nearly every night they gathered at the Super 8 to talk over the findings of the day and develop strategy. Miller realized that while Peronard's personal style wasn't exactly button-down shirts and winged-tipped shoes, his grasp of scientific methods and sampling processes were impeccable. Still, knowing that something extraordinary was happening in Libby, the team cut through as much red tape as they could. "We all went to our Rolodexes and called all the best people we knew," said Miller. "We skipped the protocols and typical chains of command because we needed answers, and we needed them quickly. We talked to all the tech and medical people we knew in government, universities, and in the private sector. We were dealing with a completely new landscape out there. Our supervisors backed us up the whole way."

During this time, the local and regional newspapers were continuing to print a number of stories on the Libby situation. The *Seattle P-I* traced the vermiculite trail throughout the country, and the *Daily Inter Lake* and the *Spokesman-Review* began to air the angry feelings of the Libby residents. Led by Benefield and Les Skramstad, a number of residents testified at a Montana Department of Environmental Quality hearing and were outspoken in their outrage against W. R. Grace. Benefield told the DEQ officials that she had complained to both the DEQ and the EPA about the mine reclamation and received no action. She told of driving to the mine site and seeing inconsistencies between the reclamation plans and what was actually at the site. She told the large crowd that she had talked to some of the men hired to do the reclamation, and although they were blasting and driving trucks and loaders across the dusty top of the mined area, the men told her they had not been warned about the asbestos danger.

A number of people testified that asbestos-related diseases were striking their families. Norita Skramstad told the crowd, "At the time my husband went to work for Zonolite, we had two small babies, two and three. And . . . forty years ago this month I had a new baby. The two older children now have it. Our youngest girl is fine, but how much longer she will be, we don't know."

Libby resident Bill Boothman said that his father, a mine employee, died of asbestosis when he was fifty-seven years old. "They said it didn't hurt him, but when I watched him die he'd hold his mouth open because he couldn't breathe, and it looked just like a bunch of maggots in there eating, on the back of his throat," Boothman testified. "And they say it didn't hurt. And now I've got it."

Libby resident Pat Vinion, who along with his two sisters has been diagnosed with advanced asbestosis, testified: "When my father was a young man they told him that you can't eat enough of that stuff. It won't bother you. Don't worry about it. Well, he's dead. When I started feeling sick when I was younger they said, 'You never worked there. It's not possible. You can't get it that way. You never worked there.' Well, it's more than possible. I am dying from it."

Peronard attended the meetings and heard the stories. "I couldn't believe it," he said. "It felt like the lining of my stomach was being ripped out."

In January 2000, the U.S. Agency for Toxic Substances and Disease Registry (ATSDR), the principal federal public health agency involved with hazardous waste issues, moved in to Libby after repeated requests by the EPA team. ATSDR was created by the Superfund law in 1980. Working with the EPA, their goal was to determine the exact extent of the public health problem in Libby. The ATSDR team, which consisted of about eight medical researchers, worked with Miller to develop a medical screening program. They began bringing residents in for chest X rays to determine how many showed the pleural thickening in their lungs that indicated asbestos exposure.

Initially, the government teams weren't sure how Libby residents would react to the free screening, and they were shocked when more than fifty-five hundred people volunteered.

Historically, government representatives, especially federal government representatives, and most especially federal government representatives from the EPA, have not found a warm welcome in Montana. Having teams from the EPA and ATSDR roaming throughout Libby normally would have caused an uproar among the local populace, but this did not happen for two reasons. The first was the ongoing series of stories in the regional newspapers reporting ATSDR findings that Libby residents were suffering sixty times more asbestos-related deaths than the rest of the country. Many of the articles were critical of W. R. Grace, which created in Libby an enemy larger even than the feds or the environmentalists.

The second reason was Peronard. He wasn't what the people of Libby expected, but he was exactly what they needed. Charismatic, credible, and always to the point, he met regularly with formal and informal residents' groups, city officials, and even representatives from Grace, and he impressed them all. Michael Jamison, a reporter for the *Missoulian* newspaper, wrote an entertaining front-page piece on Peronard, running a headline that read, EPA WITH ATTITUDE. Jamison quoted Lincoln County Commissioner Rita Windom as saying, "Paul Peronard's a bureaucrat, but he's not like any bureaucrat you've ever seen. He is more like a rock star . . . and in Libby, where he parachuted in for the EPA, he's almost as popular."

Peronard's supervisors in Denver knew they couldn't send in a guy in a three-piece suit. Still, they weren't sure how Peronard would fare. They knew he was being accepted, though, when the Denver office began receiving letters from local officials offering to foot the bill for airline tickets to fly Peronard's family from Denver to join him in Libby.

"I know the reputation Montana has for being antigovernment, but I really didn't expect any trouble," Peronard said. "We were up there to help. If you're straight with people and you're there every day, it works out."

Early on, Peronard and the EPA team established a working relationship with the W. R. Grace representatives in Libby. Although the mine had closed in 1990, Alan Stringer, the former manager of the mine during most of the 1980s, still staffed a W. R. Grace office in Libby, not far from the small office the EPA and ATSDR had leased on Mineral Avenue next to the Libby Café. Grace made headlines by promising to pay for the medical costs of everyone who suffered from asbestos-related diseases caused by the mining and expanding operations. The company also pledged $250,000 annually to the community health care center. It seemed like a large sum until people began to realize that the cost of medical care for one asbestos disease victim typically costs up to $500,000. Grace also promised to work with the EPA to clean up the asbestos-contaminated sites around Libby.

Meanwhile, Peronard and Weis were becoming increasingly concerned about the variety of exposure pathways they were finding in and around Libby. They were finding vermiculite in several home locations: in the walls and attic, the gardens and lawns, on the driveways, and just stored in sacks and piles around the homes. Peronard and Weis also began pioneering the sampling in areas that were not traditionally tested in past asbestos investigations. He knew that asbestos is most dangerous when it is actively encountered by human activity. He rationalized that while sampling attics and walls could provide good asbestos source numbers, sampling the dust in the carpets and floors of the homes would give them better actual exposure numbers. Vacuum cleaners, for example, suck up asbestos fibers, but the fibers are so small they slip through the vacuum bags and are tossed back into the air. Even walking across an asbestos-contaminated carpet can send the fibers up into the breathing zones. Because asbestos does not decompose, the fibers remain in the carpet and can continue their airborne cycle indefinitely until they are inhaled and find a place in a human lung.

By the late spring of 2000, the relationship between W. R. Grace and the EPA had taken a decided turn for the worse. Grace's promise in December to cooperate with the EPA on the cleanup of the popping and screening plants withered by April. The company refused to sign a cleanup agreement with the EPA. William Corcoran, Grace's vice president of public affairs, told the news media that the company was afraid it would lose its "rights" if it signed the agreement. At the same time, Peronard was experiencing a pattern of noncooperation from Grace. Getting records and other information from the company that would have helped determine the exposure levels of some of the people in Libby had become extremely difficult. Stringer attended many of the town meetings and began to criticize the EPA's findings that came back with elevated fiber readings. He also questioned the team's sampling techniques.

Peronard figured Stringer was just acting on orders from headquarters, but Corcoran's reluctance to help was troubling. In the mid-1990s, Peronard had been involved in a nasty industrial cleanup in Georgia that involved illegal dumping of mercury and a number of other deadly chemicals. Corcoran had represented Allied Signal, one of a number of companies involved.

"It was a big, complicated situation involving heavy-duty cleanup of about two hundred fifty thousand cubic yards of hazardous materials," Peronard said. "All the companies involved, including Allied Signal, were extremely cooperative and we got it cleaned up. When I saw that Corcoran was involved at Libby, I figured we'd get this knocked out in no time. But, there is something about working for W. R. Grace . . . nobody cooperated with us from the start."

It seemed to Peronard that the more asbestos contamination the EPA team found, the more uncooperative Grace became. After battling Grace for months for the information, Peronard finally received records of asbestos fiber tests the company had done around Libby in the past. One showed that Grace officials knew there was a high fiber count in the running track around the baseball field as early as 1981. Studies were commissioned at that time because Grace officials were growing uneasy over the vermiculite-caused diseases that were uncovered at the Scotts plant in Ohio. They applied monitors to two runners, one running directly behind the other. They found that the first runner received what is today the outer limit for fibers in occupational work areas. The second runner received double that amount as the first runner kicked up the fibers from the track, which was made primarily of mine tailings, according to Peronard. In response to the study, Grace placed a layer of asphalt over the track. "The problem was," said Peronard, "the asphalt strip wasn't wide enough. There were tailings spilling out from under the asphalt on both sides."

Grace, meanwhile, continued to deny any responsibility for any part of the asbestos contamination. Eschenbach, Grace's director of Health, Safety, and Toxicology, told the *New York Times* that they did their best to comply with the safety standards of the day. "There is no question in my mind that if the company knew how to do it, if anybody knew how to do it, it was done," Eschenbach said. "Sure, the state would come in and tell us to do more. But do what? The technology wasn't always there. If it was, we'd have used it."

By July 2000, the relationship between Grace and the EPA had deteriorated further. Grace challenged the EPA's test sampling methods, not only in Libby but also at the various vermiculite-processing plants that were being studied throughout the United States.

At one point, the EPA team had to subpoena some of Grace's records, and as Weis and Miller were going through them, they noticed that some of the files from the Libby mine were covered in dust. Weis had the dust analyzed and found it was laced with tremolite. That led to the bizarre scenario of workers in HazMat suits cleaning the company's records before they could even be reviewed.

The final straw, however, occurred in late summer, just as reports were hitting the newspapers that millions of homes may still contain contaminated vermiculite from the Libby mine. Grace reacted by denying that vermiculite was dangerous and by buying back the mine from the KDC. Immediately, Grace booted the EPA workers off the mine site where cleanup was under way.

At issue, according to Grace, was possible contaminated material that the EPA planned to dump back in the mine. The EPA had decided that rather than create a new, hazardous landfill somewhere near Libby, they would simply dump the contaminated soil and material from the screening and popping plants and the town itself back into the mine. The plan was to ultimately cover and cap the contaminated mine.

The problem focused on the twenty-one-acre site that once housed the screening plant. Grace had sold it in 1993 to Libby residents Mel and Lerah Parker, who developed it into a commercial nursery. The Parkers were aware at the time that there were legal actions being brought against Grace for mine contamination, but they said no one from Grace told them the site they bought was also contaminated.

The Parkers had established a thriving nursery, complete with greenhouses that contained large fans for ventilation. In 1994, and again in 1996, the EPA received letters from an unnamed Libby resident warning that the site was grossly contaminated with asbestos fibers. The letters also warned that Rainy Creek Road was heavily contaminated. The logging trucks that roared up and down the road kicked up barrels of dust every day that settled on the Parkers' property. Both complaints turned out to be true. In a 2001 report by the EPA's Office of Inspector General, the agency admitted it did nothing in response to the letters other than refer them to the State of Montana, which also did not investigate. The situation was ignored until Peronard found highly elevated levels of amphibole asbestos fibers throughout the former screening plant area. The Parkers had no choice but to leave their contaminated home and belongings behind and move off the property. Mel and Lerah Parker have since been diagnosed with abnormalities on their lungs.

Peronard ordered a $3 million cleanup of the former screening site, but Grace officials stopped the project by barring the agency from the mine. In a letter to the Libby Citizen Advisory Group, Stringer explained the company's reason. "First, there is the question of what, if any, chemicals contaminate the soil the EPA proposes to dump at the former mine site," he wrote. "Since the screening property was a working nursery for the last six years, we assume that some horticultural chemicals were spilled and soaked into the soil. . . . This is an important issue because the danger exists that these chemicals could find their way into the local waters. I hope we can agree that nobody wants that to happen."

The company also seemed to take a sudden interest in the safety of the workers doing the cleanup. "We must know who is responsible for the safety of the workers moving the dirt," Stringer wrote.

The letter outraged many Libby residents, as well as the EPA team. That Grace would suddenly show great concern about the harmful effects of pollution seemed hypocritical at best. Peronard saw it as just another attempt by the company to obstruct the EPA's effort to clean up the problem.

"At that point, we knew that the relationship between us and Grace, which had been problematic already, was going to be a straight fight," he said. "They weren't being difficult anymore, they were being impossible."

Not long afterward, the situation between Grace and the EPA became personal. It started when the ATSDR released the results of a preliminary medical screening, shocking the town and the EPA team.

"I was in the Denver office in a meeting when a conference call from the ATSDR team in Libby came in," said Peronard. "They gave the numbers to us, and we felt sure they were making a mistake. They talked in this monotone—totally unexcited—and we knew they had to be making a mistake. When they faxed us the report, I felt like I had been kicked in the stomach. Nearly twenty percent of the people tested had abnormal lung X rays, which meant they had an asbestos-related disease. We were stunned. We looked at each other in total disbelief. It had to be an error."

It wasn't. In fact, the number reflected the percentage of X rays that were labeled as "abnormal" by two "B-readers," expert radiologists. Up to 30 percent of the X rays were labeled abnormal by at least one B-reader. Among the former mine workers at Libby, more than 48 percent had abnormal X rays. One former Grace employee pointed out that it turned out to be more dangerous for the men to work at the mine than it was for the soldiers in WWII to land on Normandy beach against heavy enemy fire.

No one on the EPA or ATSDR teams had ever experienced such widespread poisoning before, especially in a group of people who did not work directly with asbestos. Peronard, Weis, and Miller

feared the percentage of lung abnormalities would hold for the other
seven thousand people in the Libby area who had not yet been
tested. The screening results were front-page news in every newspaper in the region. For many residents, it was the first time they
learned of the full scope of the contamination. Entire families were
found to be sick. In one family, eight children, plus the parents, had
serious lung abnormalities.

Those diagnosed were angry, frustrated, and terrified. An asbestos support group established in Libby was filled to the limit
practically overnight and had to be closed to new participants due
to lack of funding.

Soon after the preliminary test results were released, Stringer
appeared on a local radio program to protest the findings. He argued that it was irresponsible to release such preliminary data and
questioned the veracity of the test.

At one of the next Citizen Advisory Group meetings, a tape of
Stringer's interview was played. A fistfight nearly ensued when
Peronard heard Stringer refer to those with lung abnormalities as
"alleged victims."

"It was infuriating to hear him say that," Peronard said. "I was
sitting there, and I almost came out of my chair. I said, 'Alan, I can't
believe that Grace pays you enough to say that.'" Peronard followed
up with some other, more colorful words, and the point was made.
Grace's cavalier attitude was not going unchallenged.

Grace responded by increasing its resistance to the EPA's effort.
"They gave us all kinds of misdirection, they complained to Congress, they wanted us all removed from the site," said Peronard.
"They agreed to deals with us and then changed their minds. They
attacked our sampling methods and told us there was no medical
problem in Libby, and that we didn't need to clean up the high
school track because they had put down asphalt. They flat lied to us
several times."

As the scope of the project continued to expand, asbestos contamination was found at the middle and elementary schools, and more homes and gardens were found to be contaminated. It was alarming to all the government teams that many people who had never been to the mine, or had asbestos in their homes, had lung abnormalities. Dust from the mine and the popping plant was blamed in these cases.

The EPA team realized with dismay that every child who ever played on the Libby baseball fields, whether from Troy, Kalispell, or Bonners Ferry, was potentially exposed.

Meanwhile, the estimated cleanup bill kept escalating, reaching now into the tens of millions of dollars, and Grace remained uncooperative. In September, the EPA struck back. The agency filed suit against Grace to gain access to the mine. The agency won the court battle, and Grace had to unlock the gates. The EPA continued using the mine as a depository for the waste dirt and vermiculite they found at the screening and expanding plants, the schools, and throughout the rest of Libby.

When the national media suddenly found its way to Libby, Benefield, Skramstad, Wilkins, and other troublemakers made the most of it. Benefield appeared in a *People Magazine* article entitled "The Avenger," and Skramstad was featured in a piece in *Men's Journal*. Wilkins and others were interviewed a number of times as the media from the *New York Times* to National Public Radio covered the tragedy in Libby.

"It was the only chance we had of leveraging power against Grace," said Skramstad. "This was still a big, powerful company we were fighting, and we still weren't winning."

Grace's stock in Libby took another severe downturn in late September when the *Montanian* newspaper broke a story involving a New Jersey woman who said she had sat in on private meetings with Peter Grace and other executives in 1982 when they talked about establishing an "accrual fund" to pay settlements to the families of Grace workers in Libby, whom they expected to die of asbestos-related diseases.

"There were major accruals that were set up in the hundreds of millions of dollars for the possibility of lawsuits against W. R. Grace & Company from people who were going to contract a disease that would lead to their death as a result of exposure to asbestos," Lynn Latchford told the *Montanian*. Latchford said she worked as a financial analyst at Grace headquarters, which was then in New York City.

Latchford told the newspaper that she quit her job soon afterward. "It made me very angry when W. R. Grace had perpetrated not just this but also the contamination of water wells in Massachusetts, which I was aware of when I was [working at Grace]. I quit the company . . . because it was extremely dissatisfactory to me that the company was being sued on multiple levels from multiple people and I was aware of the lawsuits and the potential harm to the health of people, and I was very upset that they were pretty much playing a numbers game with what was occurring."

As the year wore on, Libby's schools became an increasing focus for Peronard's team. Early information from Grace and other sources indicated there wasn't much of a problem, but the EPA team continued to find new sources of contamination. In talking with an older employee at Plummer Elementary School, Peronard learned that truckloads of tailings and vermiculite from the mine were once dumped into a large depression near the school. Water was then poured into the hole in the winter, and it was used as a skating rink for the entire town. When Peronard drove to the school to investigate, he saw the pit had become a playground without the ice. Two boys were wrestling around in the bottom of it when he arrived, and they were covered with dust, which was later found to be highly toxic. The bottom of the old skating rink was packed with a six-inch-thick ring of vermiculite tailings.

Other elementary schools in the area were not contaminated, but a new horror surfaced when the running track at the Libby Middle School was found to be nearly 100 percent vermiculite tailings. It was immediately closed down, as was the high school track. Libby High School's season-opening football game that fall was re-located to Bonners Ferry, Idaho, an hour's drive away, because asbestos fibers were also found in great numbers under the bleachers, in the press box, and in the concession stand. The school sites had asbestos soil contamination levels reaching from 3 to 15 percent.

Letters were sent out to residents throughout the northwestern portion of Montana, warning everyone who played at the contaminated Libby schools that they may have been exposed to a potentially lethal dust.

In late November 2000, Peronard had been in Libby for more than a year. He shook his head when he thought of Tracy's worry the year before that it might take more than a week to take care of the problem. He was about to spend his second winter in Libby, and there was no end in sight.

It was turning out to easily be the biggest and most intense project of his life. He was proud of what Weis, Miller, he, and the rest of the EPA team had managed to accomplish, especially in light of the constant opposition by Grace. There were rumors that Grace was now considering filing for Chapter 11 bankruptcy to avoid the tens of thousands of asbestos-related lawsuits. Most of the lawsuits came from Grace's sales of Monokote, but an increasing number of legal cases were stemming from the vermiculite mine. Grace had not won a single case that had gone to trial involving the mine and the pollution in Libby.

By the end of the year, the EPA team had taken more than one thousand samplings in Libby, and cleanup plans were under way for the screening plant, export plant, and schools. Libby owed a debt of gratitude to Peronard and the EPA team, as well as to Benefield, Wilkins, Skramstad, and the other troublemakers. Without their efforts, the tragedy in Libby might have remained a terrible secret, as it did in Manville, New Jersey, Tyler, Texas, and other communities plagued by asbestos across the country. Still, as the numbers of sick and dying people continued to grow, Libby struggled to find something to feel thankful about.

12

WHY ASBESTOS REMAINS AMERICA'S MOST LETHAL SECRET

"The EPA has taken the lead in zero-tolerance policies to-ward any 'carcinogenic' substance . . . [including] asbestos. This draconian approach has served to encourage un-founded health scares, and created an environment in which people no longer make rational decisions about health risks."

—*editorial in the* Wall Street Journal, *April 5, 2002*

"I don't believe the Wall Street Journal *has ever been to Libby, Montana."*

—*rebuttal by Bob Wilkins, June 29, 2002*

Despite the devastation its fibers have already caused, and the substantial health threat they continue to pose, asbestos remains an invisible killer. Even recent news coverage of the events in Libby and the potential asbestos contamination from the World Trade Center haven't really dented the American consciousness. Arsenic, lead, and other chemicals are on the American radar screen, but asbestos is not. To the public and most governmental regulatory agencies and politicians, it remains a problem of the past.

"That attitude just doesn't make sense to me," said Paul Peronard. "I've dealt with all types of toxic chemicals, and asbestos is by far the more prevalent and dangerous. It is a huge problem. Why this isn't a top health priority, and why we aren't spending millions of dollars on asbestos before we spend money on lead in soils or arsenic in the water are things I don't understand. There isn't a rational explanation for it."

Peronard, of course, is speaking from the position of knowledge about asbestos that few other people in the country possess. The problem is that the truth about asbestos has been slow to reach the American public. The most obvious reason for that is the successful cover-up by the asbestos industry of the dangers of the manufacture and use of its products. It is a strategy that includes the publishing of untruths, half-truths, and misleading information regarding its product. For example, the asbestos industry, which still promotes and defends its primary product, chrysotile, continues to use the dangers of the other types of asbestos (called amphiboles), such as that found in Libby and elsewhere, as a promotable villain. Industry supporters have continued to float the concept that it is the amphibole contamination in chrysotile that causes human health problems, not chrysotile itself. The fact is that few nonindustry experts today believe that pure chrysotile is not a toxin.

The Asbestos Institute continues to make outrageous and misleading claims such as this one on their Web site: "Workers in this industry, whether employed in the manufacture, installation or removal of materials, are not exposed to any detectable risk when effective prevention and control measures are applied." The problem with that grandiose announcement is that neither the industry nor the government has proved reliable when it comes to providing and enforcing "effective prevention and control measures." Moreover, removal and abatement companies—although some clearly do the job correctly—are notorious for evading safety and training regulations. The institute's claim conveniently ignores these realities.

The institute's Web site also states, "Banning chrysotile-cement [the number one product made of chrysotile] will not resolve the problem of friable insulation in buildings. It may, however, contribute to unwarranted public paranoia and a rush to initiate unnecessary and potentially dangerous removal work."

This statement is as insulting as it is ridiculous. No one argues that banning asbestos will solve the tremendous problem now facing us with the millions of tons of asbestos that remain in millions of homes and buildings in the United States. Banning it will, however, keep the problem from expanding and extending even further into future generations. The industry shoots itself in the foot with the statement that friable asbestos in buildings is indeed a "problem." If it poses such a health risk, why should we place even more of it in our homes, office buildings, and schools?

At the same time, the institute seeks to save us from ourselves and keep us from falling into a state of "unwarranted paranoia." The fact is, once it is provided the correct information about a threat, the American public typically acts quickly to confront and eliminate the problem. That is precisely why the industry has worked so hard over the years to keep that information out of the hands of workers and consumers.

More disturbing has been the role of the regulatory agencies of the federal and state governments. The EPA has said many times that it "dropped the ball" in Libby. The State of Montana has been more circumspect about the multiple errors it made in Libby because it faces a series of lawsuits over the issue. Clearly, however, the regulatory agencies, whose job it is to protect the American public from occupational and environmental hazards, rate an "F" for the job they have done in the past in terms of regulating asbestos. The EPA did make occasional attempts to deal with asbestos, such as its ill-fated ban in 1989, but its efforts were sporadic at best. The U.S. Navy, too, rates a failing grade for not protecting its workers in the shipyards.

Today, most state and federal agencies remain woefully behind in their knowledge about asbestos. Many state asbestos coordinators still quote the old, errant myths. The chief of environmental health in one Midwestern state said emphatically in early June of 2002 that "the only true hazards from asbestos are to those who deal with it occupationally." Another state asbestos coordinator said, with equally unfounded confidence, that "air sampling is not necessary when you are testing for asbestos. The standard way is to do a visual." When he was informed that asbestos fibers are microscopic in size, he suddenly had to take another phone call.

More than a dozen federal, state, and local officials, each of whom has regulatory jurisdiction over asbestos contamination in one form or another, provided erroneous information during interviews.

Although the EPA has taken the lead on asbestos research and enforcement, its efforts are often hampered and victimized by politics. For example, the EPA Web site states that there is "no safe level of asbestos." Then, without any acknowledgment of the contradiction, it proceeds to outline the governmental regulation that states that if there is less than 1 percent asbestos in a product, that product is not considered to contain asbestos. The "1 percent rule" came about not because a product containing less than 1 percent asbestos is "safe," but because of the limitations of the optimal microscopy. Despite the development of the more powerful transmission electron microscopy (TEM) instruments, the EPA has not changed this regulation.

Few experts believe that the OSHA threshold level of asbestos fibers in the workplace protects workers. "The level that OSHA set— 0.1 fiber per cubic centimeter—was a compromise between business and health experts," Peronard said. "It is a ratio of death to dollars. It allows workers to breathe millions of fibers per day."

Research done by NIOSH states unequivocally that the OSHA level is not protective. Despite the NIOSH finding, the U.S. Mine Safety and Health Administration set its asbestos fiber level at 0.2 fibers per cubic centimeter, which is twice as high as the unsafe OSHA standards. "Right now we don't have a system that works," said Peronard. "We have set up a situation that guarantees that people are going to get sick."

Over the years, the media, too, have contributed greatly to the public's confusion about asbestos. The story of its dangers, and the wake of death it has left behind, has largely been missed by most of the national media. Much of the coverage that did take place in the past few decades was filled with inaccuracies.

Even today, it is not unusual to see articles in major publications that refer to asbestos as a "banned substance" or that echo as gospel the industry line that a little asbestos won't hurt you. The conservative, business-oriented magazines lead the way, using industry-borrowed expressions like "asbestos panic attack" and the "needless national hysteria" over asbestos. Some of this attitude was the result of the suppression of the truth about asbestos fibers by the industry, but further bias has emerged as the parent companies of many of the primary media outlets have come under fire from asbestos plaintiffs. As the number of asbestos lawsuits has skyrocketed in recent years, so too has the number of defendant companies,

many of which purchased smaller companies that once made asbestos products. Almost across the board, those magazines, newspapers, and television stations that are owned by conglomerates
being sued have begun to run editorials that read as though they
were fashioned by the asbestos industry.

Many of those without the legal entanglements avoid reporting
on asbestos because it, like a number of environmental subjects, has
become politically incorrect. The bombast of conservative radio
shock jocks like Rush Limbaugh has presented asbestos concerns as
yet another form of "ecoterrorism" and made them the target of
ridicule—like global warming was until recently. It became "uncool"
even among liberals to fear asbestos.

Much of the most accurate and revealing investigative work is
being done by regional newspapers, whose parent companies are
free of the asbestos litigation. Reporters like Bill Burke, Kevin Carmody, Michael Hawthorne, Lynette Hintze, and Andrew Schneider
have done exemplary work, but their newspapers have limited cir-
culations. Of the large-circulation publications, the *New York Times*
and the *Los Angeles Times* have provided accurate coverage in recent years.

These writers are up against impressive foes, however. For
decades, the asbestos industry has employed some of the most ex-
pensive and powerful public relations firms in America. In 1992,
Alicia Mundy wrote an article titled "Is the Press Any Match for
Powerhouse P.R.?" in the prestigious *Columbia Journalism Review*.
In it, she wrote that:

"An inside look at a 'classic propaganda campaign' by [public
relations giant] Hill and Knowlton was recently provided by *The
Daily Record*, a business and legal newspaper in Maryland, in the
form of a memorandum—one of several confidential documents
released in court as the result of a lawsuit over the installation of asbestos in public buildings in Baltimore." Mundy pointed out that

while the memo was drawn up in 1983, the PR strategy in it is time-less. She wrote: "Representing U.S. Gypsum, which for years had used asbestos in some products, H&K advised Gypsum that 'the spread of media coverage must be stopped at the local level and as soon as possible.' One focus of this strategy was to plant stories in op-ed pages 'by experts sympathetic to the company's point of view.' The plan included placing articles attesting to the safety of as-bestos."

Mundy's article goes on to say that Gypsum implemented the strategy and got favorable op-ed pieces printed in Baltimore and De-troit. The company's public relations consultant actively fed propa-ganda to a "special writer," who planted it as often as he could.

Mundy also wrote that an interoffice Gypsum memo recom-mended that the company set up a special team to "take the heat from the press and industry critics" and suggested that Gypsum should enlist scientists and doctors as "independent experts" to counter claims that asbestos is a health risk. "It can then position the problem as a side issue that is being seized on by special interests and those out to further their own causes," the twenty-five-page memo continued. "The media and other audiences important to U.S. Gypsum should ideally say, 'Why all this furor being raised about this product? We have a non-story here.'"

The company stood to benefit not only by influencing the public but also by having the industry-designed information find its way into court exhibits and perhaps sway juries. H&K execu-tives told Mundy that the strategy outlined in the 1983 memo was "old-fashioned," but Mundy could have written that same article today. Recent op-ed pieces appearing in *Time*, the *Wall Street Journal*, and *Fortune* were little more than public relations pieces for companies being sued by asbestos plaintiffs, which is fair enough, considering they were in the editorial section. The in-triguing thing to note, however, is how faithfully the asbestos sup-

porters have followed the strategy laid down for them by PR consultants twenty years ago.

The industry, when faced with a critical article on asbestos, was
also advised to "attack any and all flaws in a reporter's story, then use
them to discredit the whole piece," according to Mundy. The public
relations companies' philosophy, "as summed up by clients, is: if you
get them to back down on minor details they've screwed up on,
they're unlikely to fight you on the major ones."

Myriad other reasons have also come together to keep asbestos out
of the public eye. The long latency period is primary among them.
It takes so long for a person to get sick after being exposed that the
dramatic impact of an immediate cause and effect is lost. Plus, as
Peronard pointed out, most of the victims have been older men,
perhaps the most "expendable" people in our society. We have long
accepted that a percentage of blue-collar male workers will die
from occupational diseases. The long latency period of asbestosis,
lung cancer, and mesothelioma—and the fact that most of these
men "die quietly"—only adds to their nearly invisible status in our
communities. Moreover, many were immigrants who felt lucky to
be in America and luckier still to have a job. Their lives in America
were far better compared to the conditions they or their parents
had known in their home countries. Few were willing to file complaints with the regulatory agencies or go to the media to complain
about companies that were willing to keep them employed for
years.

Supposed objective international research has also added to the
sea of misinformation about asbestos. Asbestos industry supporters
and employees have long infiltrated and exerted strong influence on
the findings of international bodies such as the World Health Orga-

nization (WHO) and the International Program on Chemical Safety (IPCS), a program located at WHO headquarters in Geneva, Switzerland. According to an article written by Barry Castleman and Dr. Richard Lemen, a former U.S. assistant surgeon general, in the *International Journal of Occupational and Environmental Health*, representatives from chemical and asbestos companies have not only intensely lobbied international organizations, they have been instrumental in shaping policy and "scientific" findings for several years. In the past decade, many individuals and organizations, such as NIOSH, have begun to heavily criticize the undue industry influence. A rebellion of eighty-one scientists in 1996, who wrote strongly worded letters to the United Nations and other international groups, caused some of the key industry supporters to step down from their leadership positions in the IPCS and other international organizations, according to Castleman and Lemen.

Other supposedly objective international organizations, such as the International Fiber Safety Group, were exposed as industry fronts. The organization, which hoped to hold asbestos training workshops in Brazil and Mexico, was actually created by the international asbestos industry.

In the past few years, organizations like the Collegium Ramazzini, an international group dedicated to banning asbestos worldwide that is headed by Dr. Philip Landrigan of Mount Sinai Hospital and includes some of America's other top physicians and asbestos experts, have gained a much greater voice in the international community.

The reason this fight is so critical is the findings of these international organizations are often taken as gospel by countries that do not have the resources to make these studies on their own. Castleman and Lemen warned that biased scientific findings by these organizations can be "used to both misinform developing countries and to overturn worker and environmental protection measures in the industrialized world."

A final reason that asbestos has remained in the shadows of our national consciousness is that asbestos-related diseases have yet to find a sympathetic spokesperson. This is critical because it has escaped our national focus and has therefore not received any appreciable state and federal research funds. The same was true for breast cancer research years ago before women like Betty Ford began to speak out about the dangers of the disease. Today, actors, politicians, athletes, and other celebrities champion a variety of diseases and help bring them to the attention of the public and, ultimately, Congress. To date, that has not happened for asbestos-related diseases.

Besides Steve McQueen, three of the most famous victims of asbestos are U.S. Navy admiral Elmo Zumwalt, scientist Stephen Jay Gould, and Minnesota congressman Bruce Vento. Zumwalt's death was especially poignant given the ironies of his career. He took over the helm of the navy in 1970, a time when asbestos was still being used on navy ships, despite the widespread knowledge of its dangers. During the admiral's time in power, official asbestos-related deaths in shipyard workers rose to more than twenty-four hundred per year, and most experts feel that the real number was far higher.

From 1968 to 1970, Zumwalt also served as commander of the American naval forces in Vietnam, and he ordered the spraying of the defoliant Agent Orange in the Mekong Delta. One of the boats patrolling the Delta was commanded by his son, Lieutenant Elmo Zumwalt III. When cancer, which both the father and the son attributed to Agent Orange, claimed the life of his son at age forty-two, it brought about a cathartic change in the admiral.

Once a proponent of extensive chemical use, he began to lobby Congress relentlessly to provide funding for research into the cancers caused by Agent Orange and other chemicals. He explained to his family and others that he had checked with the chemical companies before he used Agent Orange and was reassured that it was "safe."

What the admiral didn't know at the time was that he was slowly dying from cancer caused by another product that the industry has long promised is "safe." In 1999, doctors found a tumor on his left lung, and he was diagnosed with mesothelioma. A tracheotomy left him unable to speak and when he died months later, a potentially powerful voice against the disease was silenced forever. Another son, James Zumwalt, has publicly denounced the industry. He told news reporters, "The asbestos companies had known of the problems for more than a half a century. They exposed thousands and thousands of people. It was absolutely inexcusable."

Stephen Jay Gould, one of the most famous scientists of the twentieth century, died of mesothelioma in 2002. Unfortunately, though he was outspoken about his views on evolution and other scientific matters, Gould was reticent when it came to discussing the disease that killed him. While his modesty was the measure of his personal warmth and the high quality of his life, it did not serve to help publicize the disease. Gould, who won dozens of scientific awards during his lifetime and served as the president of the American Association for the Advancement of Science from 1999 to 2000, was diagnosed with mesothelioma in 1982. The disease usually claims its victims about eight months after diagnosis, yet Gould fought it for more than twenty years.

The closest Gould came to making a public statement on mesothelioma came in an essay he wrote for a 1985 issue of *Discover Magazine*. It was a touching look at a man staring death in the face, but typically, he covered his true feelings with humor and saw it all with an objective, scientific eye. Gould wrote: "The literature couldn't have been more brutally clear: mesothelioma is incurable, with a median mortality of only eight months after discovery. I sat stunned for about 15 minutes, then smiled and said to myself: so that's why they don't give me anything to read."

Gould's essay then wound through the mathematics of the probability that he would survive beyond the eight-month median of mesothelioma victims. While intellectually stimulating, it was not the type of article likely to inspire a made-for-television movie or big-screen film, which is often the primary way, these days, to put a disease and corporate malfeasance on the map. (Asbestos-related disease victims are waiting for an *Erin Brockovich* or *A Civil Action* type of film to be made on the intrigues of the asbestos industry.)

Still, Gould's essay reveals the enormous heart and soul of a man who fought the deadly cancer and became one of the longest-lived mesothelioma victims on record. "It has become, in my view, a bit too trendy to regard the acceptance of death as something tantamount to intrinsic dignity," Gould concluded. "Of course, I agree with the preacher of Ecclesiastes that there is a time to love and a time to die—and when my skein runs out I hope to face the end calmly. For most situations, however, I prefer the more martial view that death is the ultimate enemy—and I find nothing reproachable in those who rage mightily against the dying of the light."

Congressman Vento, a twelve-term Democrat from Minnesota, died of mesothelioma in October 2000. Like Gould, Vento was an accomplished but also modest man. He felt it would have been self-serving to talk about his disease and suffering, and he kept it almost entirely to himself.

Vento was best known as a champion of the environment. He served as the chairman of the Subcommittee on National Parks, Recreation and Public Lands before he left Congress due to his illness. He helped pass hundreds of laws protecting the environment, including some that clamped a tighter lid on airborne toxins. He was well aware of the irony of an advocate of clean-air issues being struck down by a cancer caused by an airborne contaminate. Vento blamed his exposure on jobs he had as a laborer when he was young.

Vento's death was not an easy one. He lost a lung and his diaphragm to surgeries and underwent three cycles of chemotherapy only to have the tumors come back. Before he died, he took issue with the Bush administration's termination of his grant to continue research into the genetic basis for mutations that give rise to mesothelioma cells. It was a particularly bitter blow to Vento, delivered by a president whose father had refused to stand up for the EPA's ban on asbestos in 1989. Today, none of the more than $20 billion of the National Cancer Institute's budget is being applied to mesothelioma research, according to the Mesothelioma Applied Research Foundation (MARF), the private consortium of physicians trying to fight the disease.

Vento, who was a junior high science and social studies teacher before he ran for Congress in 1976, was one of the more respected members of Congress.

On a night honoring Vento in Washington, D.C., President Clinton praised him by calling him a caring man "who never stopped being a teacher. . . . Tonight, as he fights a disease that has not yet yielded all its secrets to science, he's our teacher again." Clinton's words were the only mention of his disease that night.

While such stoicism is absolutely admirable from a personal standpoint, present and future asbestos-related disease victims need passion and noise and perhaps even outrageousness from victims in order to focus America's attention. What mesothelioma victims need is not a heroic Gary Cooper, but a raucous Erin Brockovich. Future asbestos victims desperately need "those who rage mightily against the dying of the light."

13

A TOWN DIVIDED

"It would have been more honorable for a person to take a gun and rob a bank than to do what that company did to this town."

—Jim Racicot

The Dome Theater, Libby's only movie house, sits just a few blocks south of Paul Peronard's EPA office on Mineral Avenue. Painted on the outside of the small, thin building, where the ticket cashier sits behind a tiny glass window that conjures up images of the 1950s, is a mural of a small boy carrying an American flag. A huge grizzly bear rears up in the background. The words above the boy read "God Bless America."

The Dome doesn't always get first-run movies, but it usually gets them before they arrive in the ubiquitous movie rental outlets around town. On weekends, acting troupes from around Montana put on plays there, which are often sold out weeks ahead of time. Being literally the only show in town, the Dome Theater is usually a busy place.

It was no surprise, though, that it was nearly deserted the week that the film *A Civil Action* came to town. John Travolta's hip and poignant portrayal of Boston attorney Jan Schlichtmann, who had sued W. R. Grace and others over the pollution-caused deaths of several children near Woburn, Massachusetts, did not amuse many residents. The film was not flattering to Grace and although there was no organized boycott, it did not play well in western Montana. Despite everything that had happened, Libby was still a company town.

By the spring of 2001, however, Libby's story began to find legs in the regional and national media. Benefield, Wilkins, Skramstad, and some of the other Libby victims—most of whom had never talked to a reporter in their lives—gave dozens of interviews. It was a time when they should have felt a sense of satisfaction that their stories were finally being told and the dangers of asbestos were being revealed. Benefield was fulfilling the promise that she had made to her mother, and Wilkins and Skramstad were exposing the betrayal of their employers. But instead, the Libby troublemakers were finding that the story was far from over. And their frustrations were greater than ever.

Grace continued to deny responsibility for the town's contamination. The company drew a line in the sand and was planning to fight the troublemakers as well as Peronard and the EPA at every turn. The company also was refusing to pay for the cleanup, arguing that it had done what it could to protect the town and the miners. Tensions on both sides mounted as the cleanup costs soared.

"It was an intensely difficult time," said Peronard. "We felt pressure from the community because we still had to clean up the schools and some of the other public areas. Beyond that, we knew we still had a serious problem with the homes in the area. People were still living in houses that were full of vermiculite. With every day that went by, these folks faced the potential of additional asbestos exposure."

The constant pressure of dealing with Grace, with the outcomes often becoming front-page headlines, took its toll on Peronard. Wilkins, Benefield, and others feared he might be fired or transferred by the EPA, but the agency stuck by him. The worst part of all for Peronard was the fact that many of the people he had come to know in Libby were dying or already dead.

During one of his infrequent trips back to Denver to spend time with his family, he complained of stomach problems to his wife, Tracy. A trip to his doctor confirmed that he had developed an ulcer.

Ironically, even as Peronard's team and the other governmental health agencies gained widespread respect and acceptance in Libby, a bitter divide was growing within the community itself. The troublemakers were finding that not only was Grace opposing them, so was much of the rest of the town.

The division in Libby was due less to the town's blind loyalty to Grace than it was a desperation born out of suffocating fear that the already mean economic times in Libby could get worse. Unemployment hovered near the 15-percent mark, and most of the jobs that were available paid little more than minimum wage. Libby, for all the natural, awe-inspiring splendor of the surrounding wilderness, suffered the similar economic convulsions as many inner-city areas in America. People wanted to work but there were few jobs available. In Libby, many of those out of work were too proud to go on welfare. Out of desperation, they often took part in a subterranean cottage industry called "horn hunting." They combed the forest for antlers shed by elk, deer, and moose and sold them to tourist shops, hoping the money would get them through until they could find a job. Anyone who threatened the fragile economy of the area—no matter how justifiable their cause—was bound to make bitter enemies.

"You can imagine a small town in Montana finding all its problems featured in the *New York Times*," said Peronard. "There was a deer-in-the-headlights effect. The people here didn't like it. It seemed like the nation was being told that Libby was a dying town full of poison. Home sales are down because of the bad press coverage. It was tough for people here to handle."

The bitterness cost Bob Wilkins his best friend. "We had worked at the mine together and had been like brothers for twenty-five years," Wilkins said. "He was a pallbearer in my wife's funeral. But from the day he learned I was sick, his attitude changed toward me. One day he looked away and said that anyone who would file a lawsuit against Grace was nothing but a freeloader. Well, I told him I'd be happy to give him everything I got in the settlement if he would give me his good lungs. We don't talk anymore."

From the beginning, Gayla Benefield was the most outspoken of the "troublemakers." She harangued bureaucrats, politicians, and even doctors who refused to diagnose asbestos as a cause of illness and death in Libby. She kept up on every issue involving Grace and the cleanup, and made sure the company was sticking by its promises to help those who were sick. She was relentless, even in the face of sometimes-bitter criticism by some of the town's business leaders.

"The town hated me at first," she said. "I don't know of another way to put it. The business people and the real estate agents and nearly everyone else feared we were scaring away tourists and people who wanted to buy property up here. They wanted us to shut up about the contamination. They said there wasn't a problem. They blamed the media for blowing it out of proportion. We had hundreds of people dying up here and they said it was all rumors."

At first, Benefield was the lone voice of complaint against Grace in the Citizen Advisory Group. The CAG had been formed to provide a liaison between the community and the EPA and other agencies. The group's recommendations usually made front-page news in the region, and they were posted on the Internet and scrutinized by asbestos activists worldwide. The meetings were often testy, full of glowering looks and insinuations that Benefield should go home and keep her mouth shut. She did neither. Sometimes she fought so hard that the line blurred between friends and enemies.

"Goddamn, you have to take your hat off to her," said Jim Racicot. "She can be abrasive and obnoxious at times, but she's run into a brick wall so many times she's calloused up."

These were difficult times for Benefield, but the memory of her parents stiffened her resolve. She could never forget the disillusionment and pain of her father's last days, or the bitterness and anger on her mother's face. It also appeared their deaths were only the beginning. The Agency for Toxic Substances and Disease Registry (ATSDR) screening revealed that Gayla herself had fibrosis in her lungs. More than thirty members of her extended family were also diagnosed with lung abnormalities caused by the tremolite fibers. In the spring of 2001, Benefield had no trouble finding motivation to fight. Still, Grace seemed to hold most of the cards, especially since the once tight-knit community had split apart.

The split between Libby's residents became starkly evident on Memorial Day 2001. Benefield had helped spearhead the planning of a dedication ceremony that included placing nearly two hundred white crosses—one for each of the known victims of the vermiculite mine—along Highway 2. The idea horrified the business community.

"When they found out I was involved, I got threats and people calling me saying they would sue me if we did this thing," said

Racicot, who helped Benefield plan the ceremony. "It was like we were going to war. I said, 'Go ahead and sue. Grace already took my health, you may as well take the rest.'"

Benefield and Skramstad were also threatened with lawsuits. Under pressure, the Libby City Council reached a compromise by allowing the memorial to be held at the Libby Cemetery, far from the highway. Still, it made the front pages of the regional newspapers and was a victory of sorts for Benefield and the troublemakers. On each cross was stenciled the name of an asbestos victim. When they were placed in the cemetery, in long rows, the result was a stunning panorama of death, a stark symbol of how many families had been devastated by the "nuisance dust" from the mine.

Although some businesses helped with the memorial service, many people in Libby simply refused to accept the fact that Grace, which had supported the community for so long with jobs, donations, and tax revenue, could be guilty of knowingly contaminating the entire town. It just didn't seem possible. Phrases like "hidden agendas" became popular among those siding against the asbestos victims. The plaintiff lawyers and the victims had "hidden agendas" to make money from Grace by making up stories about the contamination and suing the company. It was not unusual to hear talk on the sidewalks and in the small diners that "nobody is really sick, they just want free money."

Benefield, who took the brunt of much of the town's anger, had her own theory on the community's reaction. "Over the years, the town developed something like a battered spouse syndrome," she said. "Grace had a big checkbook and bought its way into the community. Whenever the community wanted something, Grace was right there with a check. But there was a cost to Grace's generosity. The company would be right there on the front page, giving the town fifty thousand dollars for something, while inside there would be two or three obituaries of Grace employees dying of 'lung problems' or 'emphysema.' Grace donated the property for the ball fields and told the mine managers they had to be coaches; they just didn't tell anyone the fields were toxic. They put a new roof on the grandstand for free; they just wouldn't put in showers and lockers at the mine so the men wouldn't bring home the dust. There was always this terrible trade-off."

In April 2001, the W. R. Grace Company, after more than 150 years of operation, filed for protection from its creditors under Chapter 11 of the bankruptcy code. More than 124,000 claims had been filed against the company, most of them involving the sale of the fireproofing spray Monokote. The Grace filing angered the asbestos victims, who saw it as nothing more than a way for the company to escape paying for the health and cleanup costs in Libby and the other areas it had polluted across the nation.

The pro-Grace faction argued that it was an honorable company forced into bankruptcy by greedy plaintiff lawyers. One real estate agent raised in Libby wrote a guest editorial for the Spokane *Spokesman-Review* in August 2001 titled "It's in No One's Best Interest to Beat Up on Grace." The editorial praised the jobs Grace created in Libby and proclaimed the company's innocence. The editorial stated, "Everything that was related to almost anything good in Libby is related in one way or another to the efforts of Grace. . . . Yes, some people are dying, which is very unfortunate. . . . [But] no one clearly understood the long-term implications of the problems."

Grace defended itself by pointing to the fact it had enrolled nearly two hundred people found to have abnormal lung X rays in a medical expense program, and it donated $652,000 to Libby's newly founded Center for Asbestos-Related Diseases. At the same time, Grace was paying out nearly $16 million in settlement costs re-sulting from sixty-four lawsuits filed by former miners and their families.

The pressure to downplay the widespread sickness and contamination in Libby was felt keenly inside the editorial room of the town's only newspaper, *The Western News*. "I wrote an article covering the number of people with abnormal lung X rays and some of the people in the business community got pretty mad," said publisher Roger Morris. "They were afraid it would scare outside business away. There were a number of complaints and threats. We're just a small paper. It put us in a tough position."

It wasn't the first time asbestos contamination had divided a town. Similar problems had arisen in Marysville, Ohio, and Manville, New Jersey. When Michael Hawthorne filed his stories in Marysville about the asbestos deaths caused by Libby's vermiculite at the Scotts plant, he stirred up a hornet's nest of resentment among the business community. "Nobody wanted to talk to me when I first started investigating," Hawthorne said. "It was Marysville's dirty little secret. The company ran the town. When my stories first appeared, an AM radio station said they were going to burn the newspaper in effigy in the Town Square. The company took out some very expensive ads in which they attacked me directly. They were definitely playing hardball. It was a case of the town not wanting to hear anything negative about a company that had supported it for so long."

In Manville, where the asbestos-related deaths from the Johns-Manville plant are only now beginning to decrease, no organized opposition to the deadly operations of the company ever developed. The naiveté and stoicism of the immigrant workers, the blindness of the media, and the loyalty surrounding a one-company town sup-

pressed one of the biggest stories of corporate malfeasance and occupational poisonings in American history. Even today, many
people in Manville do not harbor ill will against the company. As
one area media executive said, "People here seem to remember
Johns-Manville as a good employer and a good business for the
community." Of course, those who would disagree the loudest no
longer can.

Similarly, in Libby, although it was already known that more than
fourteen hundred residents (the number has since risen to more
than fifteen hundred) had asbestos damage to their lungs, many of
the townspeople refused to accept the problem as their own. The
"hidden agenda" references grew, and many of those who were sick,
even though they were screened and diagnosed by the ATSDR team
and local physicians, were accused of faking their illness. Some
feared economic losses from the bad publicity; others were envious
of those who had won large settlements from Grace. Many simply
didn't like hearing that their hometown was contaminated with a
deadly poison and wanted to shoot the messenger.

Bob Wilkins was one of those messengers, and a noisy one at
that. He continued to rile the businesspeople in Libby by wearing
his T-shirts that ridiculed Grace. "The whole damn town was in an
uproar," he said. "Grace ran this place for a lot of years, and now the
shit had hit the fan and everybody was up in arms. The realtors and
the business people didn't want this out. It isn't easy making a living
in Libby as it is, and now the whole nation knew we were contaminated. They used to holler at me downtown to 'Take that damn T-
shirt off!' but I never would."

Wilkins, like others who won settlements against Grace, was
forced to deal with the jealousy and spite of those who felt he was an

opportunist. "I had guys in town tell me I was looking to get something for nothing. Well, I have less than forty percent of my lungs
left and I lose more every month. I can't walk fifty feet to take the
damn garbage out without stopping to get air. I told them, 'I want
you to do me a favor. I want you to come visit me when I die. I want
you to see how I die, and afterwards I want you to come to my funeral and look into my casket, and I want you to tell me that I got
something for nothing.'"

The psychological battles faced by victims of asbestos are varied and
complex. When told they have an incurable illness, most advance
through the difficult stages of denial, anger, acceptance, and resig-
nation. The anger is accentuated for those who see their exposure as
due to a deliberate act, and it is increased exponentially by a community and political and legal systems that seemingly were unwilling
to help them find justice.

"The latency period of the disease is a big reason why people
get away with having such unjust attitudes," said Mike Powers, who
has lung abnormalities that have been traced to the vermiculite in
his house, once owned by Edward Alley, the founder of the Libby
mine. "If this was the Ebola virus or smallpox, no one could deny
the problem. But because we have something rotting away our lungs
that you can't see on the outside, they can say anything they want to.
It makes me mad as hell."

Jim Racicot still gets angry when the topic of Grace comes up.
"The company came in as a benefactor and said, 'We'll take your fathers, and if they'll pay no attention to this nuisance dust and work
hard and do what we tell them, we'll make a profit and maybe your
sons or daughters can be the first in the family to go on to college,'"
he said. "What they did was take the profit, the fathers, mothers, and
the sons and daughters, too. We were all naive, we thought corpo-

rate America cared. It does care—about its stockholders and the bottom line. Whatever happens to the rest of us is just considered collateral damage."

Bob Dedrick, now an active member of the Citizen Advisory Group board, found that fighting the company, the town, and a recalcitrant political system left him near the edge of despair. "During those first couple of years I was depressed and mad all the time," he said. "We all had counseling, but it didn't do much to curb my anger. The problem was we were fighting battles that couldn't be won. We knew we couldn't win them because the town, the company, and even the government, before Peronard got here, were against us. We fought anyway, but we didn't seem to get anywhere. It was a damn frustrating feeling." Dedrick's grandson, who had played in the vermiculite piles, was diagnosed with an asbestos disease during that time.

Libby's Center for Asbestos-Related Diseases saw so many patients that coordinator Pat Cohen developed her own instant diagnostic methods. "I would look at the shoes of the men who came into the clinic," she said. "If they had slip-ons or if the laces weren't tied, I knew they probably were having serious lung problems. They didn't have the air space left in their lungs to bend over. I would ask the women, 'Who makes your bed?' If they said someone else made it, it was usually because they have asbestosis and reaching over to spread the sheets expels too much oxygen from their lungs. It may not be scientific, but it is a reality of life here in Libby."

Helen Clarke, the clinic's outreach coordinator, found that the worst psychological burdens were carried by those men who brought the dust home with them from the mine and contaminated their families. "Even though the men were not told it was dangerous, they still harbor irreconcilable feelings of guilt," she said. Anger management is another big issue. "A lot of times the men whose families have been affected tell me they are about to lose it," she said. "I can only tell them that they have every right to be angry, and that anger is the normal reaction. There has been no violence against Grace that I know of. Despite the anger they feel, Montanans are among the most peaceable people in the world." The job has been wearing on Clarke, who has watched many clients and friends sicken and die. "I go home pretty bummed sometimes," she said.

As the situation in Libby became national news, the issue became a thorny one for Montana politicians. State Senator Bill Crismore initially loudly defended Grace and supported a state bill that would have restricted asbestos victims' rights. He later modified his stance, however, under a hail of angry criticism from the asbestos victims. U.S. Senator Max Baucus weighed in carefully on the side of the victims, securing $100,000 in federal funds, at one point, to continue the screening and ongoing health care in Libby. Montana governor Judy Martz, who began her term in 2001, also stepped carefully through what the elected officials feared could be a political minefield, with corporate and local business interests on one side and a number of sympathetic asbestos victims on the other.

The most political intrigue was generated by former governor Marc Racicot, who served from 1993 through 2000. Governor Racicot distanced himself completely from the plight of the asbestos victims in Libby, despite the fact that he had grown up in the town and several members of his extended family had either died or were sick from the fibers.

Racicot's position was especially tentative because he was a close friend of President George W. Bush and he was being considered for the GOP's top political post. "From a personal standpoint, Marc was devastated when he learned that I was diagnosed, along with my brothers and sister," said Jim Racicot, Marc's cousin. "But politically, Marc is a typical Republican and supports industry. The only conclusion I would have thought he would have come to is that Grace was dirty, that they knew a long time ago what they were doing in Libby was hurting people. I would have thought he could have said or done something because the company thought they could get away with it. And, well, now that I think about it, I guess they did get away with it."

In December 2001, Marc Racicot was unanimously elected chairman of the Republican National Committee.

Grace never wavered from its position that it did not act improperly. The company insisted that it bore no responsibility for what happened in Libby or, for that matter, the health problems associated with the tremolite in Monokote. In both cases, the company said it had used the best technology available at the time to minimize the health dangers of the tremolite. Grace officials also insisted that the company was cooperating fully with governmental agencies. Peronard disputed the claim. "They never cooperated with us—never," he said. "They fought us at every turn. They made issues out of everything. Their lawyers did nothing but try to obstruct us. I've never encountered anything like it before. I had one attorney from Grace say to me that there are no asbestos risks in Libby. I couldn't believe it. What he was saying was total fiction."

In the late spring of 2001, the EPA suggested that Libby was a candidate for a Superfund designation, which would commit federal money and resources to clean up the contamination. The suggestion ignited an angry debate. Business leaders feared that being a

Superfund site would scare off outside investment interests. Bene-field and the others believed it provided the only solution open to the town. And so everyone was shocked when it was revealed that Libby was already a Superfund site. The aquifer that provided the drinking water in the town had been polluted years before by local industry and the Superfund paid for a continual monitoring of the water supply. Nevertheless, the business interests in Libby remained against a second Superfund designation.

To others it appeared to be not only the best answer, but per-haps the only one. The federal government would pay to clean up the entire town, the EPA would bill Grace for the cleanup costs, and Libby could then present itself to the state and nation as a "clean" city. The problem was that Superfund sites almost always suffer an economic downturn immediately after being designated due to the acknowledgment that the area is severely polluted. Governor Martz and state environmental officials had official veto power over any Montana Superfund designation, and the governor had shown no signs of going against the wishes of the business community.

In September 2001, EPA administrator Christine Whitman vis-ited Libby and assured the community that the EPA was "in it for the long haul." She did not, however, make a full commitment to clean up the homes that contained vermiculite insulation. A month later, the community received good news when the EPA announced a settlement in its lawsuit against Grace over access to the mine. Grace agreed to provide $2.75 million in additional health benefits to the asbestos victims and pay a $71,000 civil penalty as part of the settlement.

But with hundreds of homes in Libby still contaminated with vermiculite, it was clear the town had to do something. Otherwise, thousands of people ran the risk of continued exposure in their own homes.

The asbestos victims' advocates scored a victory during the

summer by convincing the Lincoln County Commissioners to request that Governor Martz put Libby's potential Superfund designation on the fast track. Every state governor has one "silver bullet" that guarantees that one site within the state will be included on the EPA's National Priorities List for guaranteed long-term cleanup. The advocate group and the EPA team were deeply disappointed, however, when on October 11, 2001, Governor Martz rejected the commissioners' request. With the estimated abatement costs soaring to more than $100 million and little funding available to clean up the contaminated homes, the chances of Libby being cleaned up for good seemed very much in doubt.

14

TARGETING THIRD WORLD MARKETS

Even as more than thirty-five countries around the world have banned asbestos, including most of Europe and Australia, the market has skyrocketed in Third World countries. In Asia, for example, asbestos consumption almost doubled between 1970 and 1995. As a result, the United Nations estimates that roughly three million people in developing nations will die from asbestos-related diseases by the year 2030.

More than fifty billion pounds of asbestos were produced worldwide in the past decade, much of it sold to developing countries. If this trend continues, these countries will suffer accelerated death rates beginning ten to twenty years from now that will extend beyond 2030 into much of this century. Given that asbestosis and mesothelioma are brutal and incurable diseases, the sum of the worldwide human suffering will be incalculable.

Canada and Russia continue to be the world's leading asbestos exporters. Canada, which prohibits the use of most asbestos products within its own boundaries, exported an estimated 680 million pounds annually of chrysotile asbestos, but even that output is dwarfed by the 1.7 billion pounds of asbestos mined by Russia every year. Half of Russia's asbestos is exported.

The increasing number of national bans on asbestos has caused production to decrease worldwide from 8.8 billion pounds in 1990 to 4.1 billion pounds in 2001, and the more than 50 billion pounds of asbestos produced worldwide in the last decade was the lowest of any decade since 1950. The decreasing numbers are encouraging to those who favor a worldwide ban on asbestos, but the asbestos trade is far from being eradicated.

To understand what is in store for the developing countries, one simply needs to look at the status of industrialized countries where the latency period has run its course. As was noted earlier, an estimated quarter-million people are expected to die of mesothelioma in western Europe between 1995 and 2029. More Brits will die of asbestos-related diseases than were killed in combat during WWII, and the number does not include those fatalities that have been, and inevitably will be, misdiagnosed. Among men born in the 1940s in the United Kingdom, 1 out of every 150 will die of mesothelioma, according to England's Institute of Cancer Research in Sutton, Surrey.

Although these numbers are known to asbestos-producing companies, it is still being enthusiastically marketed to most countries around the world, especially developing nations hungry for new products. The Asbestos Institute boasts that an estimated sixty countries now use chrysotile cement. In the past decade, Asia has supplanted the United States and France as the Canadian chrysotile industry's biggest customer. Asbestos consumption in Thailand, for example, rose from 47 million pounds in 1970 to 361 million pounds in 1994. In India, consumption more than doubled during that time to a total of 271 million pounds.

Around the world, countries like Angola, Indonesia, Mexico, Nigeria, Egypt, Algeria, Zimbabwe, and Uruguay mine and import millions of pounds of asbestos. Those who believe that these countries properly safeguard their workers and consumers against asbestos most likely also believe in the tooth fairy.

The health impact on poor nations is likely to be especially devastating because many of those exposed will be workers and their families who already have poor diets and lack medical services. Many of these countries do not have child labor laws, and it is likely that large numbers of children and teenagers are exposed to the fibers. Experts believe that younger people are particularly vulnerable to asbestos diseases, especially mesothelioma. At the same time, the rate of asbestos disease is rapidly increasing in women worldwide as more women enter the workforce. Women are also being exposed to asbestos products inside their homes and to the dust on their husbands' work clothes. Mesothelioma rates in Australian women, for example, have tripled since 1985, according to government statistics quoted in the Sydney *Sunday Telegraph*.

Findings in Australia are helping, as they are in Libby, to correct the traditional thinking that asbestos diseases are strictly occupational in nature. Studies have revealed that up to 70 percent of the new mesothelioma rates in Australia are nonoccupationally related. Although exposure pathways are not always clear, researchers point to the fact that one in three houses built in Australia before 1982 contains asbestos. Moreover, Australia, once the world's largest producer of commercial crocidolite, often used the highly dangerous amphibole in household products. In some cases, third-generation users of the homes containing asbestos are now showing signs of exposure.

Attitudes toward asbestos vary widely around the world. Scandinavian countries, as they often do when it comes to environmental and worker safety issues, led the way by banning use of the fibers in the early 1980s. While the United States has turned a blind eye to the dangers of the product, most of the European Union, Australia, and countries like Saudi Arabia, Latvia, Chile, and Luxembourg have already banned it. Japan is considering a proposal to phase it out, and an agency of the United Nations has called for global trade restrictions on the sale of all forms of asbestos. The U.N. Chairman of the Interim Chemical Review Committee, Reiner Arndt of Germany, said it was a step toward a U.N. move to eliminate the asbestos trade worldwide. The list of countries that have banned asbestos use includes:

1983: Iceland bans most types of asbestos, updated in 1996.

1984: Norway bans asbestos, with a few exceptions, updated in 1991.

1986: Denmark bans chrysotile asbestos.

1986: Sweden introduces the first of a series of bans on chrysotile asbestos.

1988: Hungary bans amphibole asbestos.

1989: The United States bans asbestos, but the ban is overturned in 1991.

1989: Switzerland bans all types of asbestos.

1990: Austria bans chrysotile.

1991: Holland introduces a series of chrysotile bans.

1992: Finland introduces a phaseout ban on chrysotile.

1992: Italy bans chrysotile.

1993: Germany bans chrysotile, having banned amphiboles earlier.

1993: Croatia bans crocidolite and amosite.

1995: Japan bans amphiboles.

1996: France upsets Canadian suppliers by banning chrysotile.

1997: Poland bans all asbestos.

1998: Belgium bans chrysotile.

1998: Saudi Arabia bans all asbestos.

1998: Lithuania issues a phaseout ban culminating in 2004.

1999: The United Kingdom bans chrysotile.

2000: Ireland bans chrysotile.

2001: Brazil's four most populous states ban asbestos.

2001: Latvia bans asbestos.

2001: Chile bans asbestos.

2001: Argentina bans chrysotile; amphiboles banned in 2000.

2002: Spain and Luxembourg begin phaseout ban.

2002: New Zealand bans imports of raw asbestos.

2003: Australia asbestos ban takes effect.

2005: Hungary ban expected to take effect.

2005: European Union deadline for bans in Portugal and Greece.

2005: Slovak Republic, Croatia, and Hungary expected to adopt EU asbestos ban.

Most of the bans include minor exceptions. For example, in Germany, chrysotile-containing diaphragms for chlorine-alkali electrolysis in already existing installations will be allowed until 2011.

Only the United States and Canada remain as the major Western countries that have not yet made significant moves toward banning the use and trade of the deadly fibers. Canada is still deeply involved in mining and manufacturing asbestos products, and U.S. companies still sell asbestos products overseas. The reluctance of the United States to join in the push to ban asbestos has been a major obstacle to a worldwide phaseout of the mineral. Without the commitment of the American government, it is doubtful that its use in the developing countries will diminish anytime soon.

Part of the problem is that the successful propaganda that was used to market asbestos as a "safe" product in America has also been exported with similar success in developing countries. Many of the same deceptions perpetrated on American workers for decades are now being recycled. In India, for example, the workers who routinely slice open the bags of raw asbestos from Canada are rarely told of the dangers to their health. At one large, dust-filled asbestos-cement factory in Egypt, a reporter from *Egypt Today* was assured that there was no danger from the clouds of asbestos dust he saw there. The manager of the plant scooped up a dry, powdery pile of asbestos filings and dropped them into the reporter's hands. "Don't be afraid," the manager said. "It's wet. It's okay when it's wet." There were piles of asbestos waste and open bags of raw asbestos throughout the plant. "It's safe," the manager proclaimed, smiling. "We have eliminated the release of asbestos fibers into the environment." The factory annually passes the government's environmental and safety tests.

While Canada, Russia, and China lead the world in mining and producing the toxic fibers for commercial use, the United States provides its share for world consumption. In 2001, for example, the United States exported more than thirty million pounds of raw asbestos and asbestos products, most of it to developing countries, according to the U.S. Geological Survey.

The following is a look at the status of asbestos production and use in selected countries around the world:

BRAZIL: Like most developing countries, Brazilian officials have no idea how many asbestos victims already exist in the country. Although an estimated two hundred thousand workers use asbestos on their jobs in Brazil, there has been no research on asbestos diseases, and none is planned. Despite the absence of official data, a number of anti-asbestos advocacy groups have sprung up around the country. As a result, while the country itself has not banned asbestos, four of the most populated states and a number of cities and towns have outlawed its use. Much of the anti-asbestos sentiment in Brazil stems from the courageous actions of Fernanda Giannasi, an occupational health and safety engineer with the Brazilian Labor Ministry who has spearheaded efforts to ban the fibers throughout the country. Despite being physically threatened by industry supporters, Giannasi continues to work toward a total ban of asbestos in Brazil. This includes the importation of "Calidria," which is American asbestos mined in California.

THE UNITED KINGDOM: Having finally banned asbestos, England and Scotland now must face the massive health and financial problems associated with the millions of tons of asbestos the countries imported in the past seventy years. Most buildings there contain some asbestos in the form of cement products, insulation, and fireproofing material. The United Kingdom's Health and Safety Commission estimated that as many as 1.5 million workplace properties contain asbestos.

Shipyard workers in both seafaring countries are suffering high rates of asbestos diseases. Bill Speirs, general secretary of the Scottish Trade Union Congress, told the Glasgow *Herald*, "Scotland's proud heritage as a shipbuilding and manufacturing nation has, unfortunately, had a terrible downside in the thousands upon thousands of workers and their families who have suffered and died through exposure to asbestos."

Some cities are suffering exceptionally large numbers of casualties. The shipbuilding region near Clydebank, for example, has one of the highest death rates in Britain, ten times the national average per capita. Last year more than a thousand angry and frustrated Clydebank workers marched in the streets, calling for additional compensation and better health care for asbestos victims.

In the next fifty years, the health care and asbestos abatement costs in Scotland and England will skyrocket. In addition, exposure of office employees and abatement workers remains a possibility into the foreseeable future, especially if the abatement work is not done correctly. In July 2001, fifty thousand pounds of asbestos waste, including crocidolite and amosite, were illegally dumped at sites near Linthorpe, according to Laurie Kazan-Allen, director of the International Ban Asbestos Secretariat organization headquartered in London. The area was accessible to the public, possibly causing a new round of exposures. The perpetrators were not caught, and the area landowners had to pay the high price of the cleanup. In many ways, the real cost of decades of ignoring the fibers' lethal nature is about to come due in the United Kingdom.

INDIA: Few Indian asbestos workers understand the dangers presented by asbestos, and many are not properly protected. One anti-asbestos activist, Dr. T. K. Joshi, has gained international support for his efforts to convince the Indian government to ban asbestos. According to Barry Castleman, who has traveled in India studying the asbestos situation there, Dr. Joshi, the former president of the Indian Association of Occupational Health, faces a difficult battle and tensions often run high. Joshi has been threatened and bullied, but he continues to lead efforts to have it banned.

Most frightening are the reports that India now mines an estimated forty-four million pounds of tremolite asbestos. Much of the tremolite is reportedly mixed with chrysotile to manufacture water supply pipes. In addition to the interior asbestos mines, India imports about nineteen million pounds of chrysotile asbestos every year. The Indian government has been fairly active in developing vegetable fiber binding agents as alternatives to asbestos, but at the same time, it also lowered import duties for asbestos by 68 percent from 1995 to 2000, giving asbestos imports a decided boost. The asbestos industry, once owned by British and American companies, is now dominated by Indian-owned interests. The same propaganda employed by the Western companies, however, is still being used.

"There are three to five separate trade associations representing the asbestos industry in India, putting out familiar propaganda including paid ads in newspapers, [such as] 'recent reports linking the use of asbestos to health hazards have been once again clarified and set to rest,'" wrote Castleman. The industry arguments in India echo those throughout developing nations. They put forth the same self-serving and flawed reasoning that in poor countries desperate for housing and jobs, asbestos is a "critical" product. The truth, of course, is that the short-term profits garnered by the industry, which are rarely shared to any degree with the workers, will be dwarfed by the long-term health care, legal, and abatement costs borne by the workers and the government.

AUSTRALIA: Much like western Europe and the United States, Australia is now trying to cope with the enormous price of its past use of asbestos. Six Australians per day will die of asbestos diseases for the next twenty years. The country is expected to suffer nearly seventy thousand asbestos-related deaths between the years 1987 and 2010, according to Australia's National Occupational Health and Safety Commission.

After WWII, Australia began mining and importing asbestos on a massive scale, with most of the products used in the building industry. By the mid-1950s, the country was consuming more asbestos cement products per capita than any country in the world. The high rate of consumption continued into the 1960s as "fibro houses" made with substantial amounts of asbestos became highly fashionable. Mirroring the regulatory failures in Europe and

America, Australian courts have found that governmental agencies often failed to protect workers from obvious exposures. In one case involving a Melbourne-based stevedore who died of mesothelioma in 1998, the High Court of Australia accused the Australian Stevedoring Industry Authority of ignoring the dangers to the workers. During the trial, workers described conditions where they unloaded sacks of raw asbestos that often tore open and covered them with clouds of fibrous dust. The High Court found that:

> *As already indicated, the Authority ought to have known from its inspectors of the frequency with which and the degree to which waterside workers at the Port of Melbourne were exposed to asbestos. Further, it knew that exposure to asbestos dust and fibers could be injurious to health. It was in a position to know what, if any, steps employers were taking to avoid the risks posed by asbestos. And more to the point, if employers were not taking adequate measures, the Authority was in a position to take various steps . . . to control or minimize those risks.*

The Australian courts are now being challenged with scores of asbestos-related lawsuits. The government, which has been found negligent in many asbestos cases, is also struggling to own up to its responsibilities to the soaring number of victims. A paper presented at a health symposium in Denmark in 2001 ("Malignant Mesothelioma in Australia 1945–2000," J. Leigh et al.) estimated the percentage of deaths from asbestos that can be expected in certain groups. These included: Wittenoom miners and millers, 16 percent; power station workers, 12 percent; railway workers, 6 percent; navy and merchant marine personnel, 5 percent.

Although the Australian ban on asbestos will begin in 2003, more than three million pounds of asbestos, including nearly one million asbestos products, were imported into the country in 2001.

RUSSIA AND POLAND: The fates of these two countries are tightly bound when it comes to asbestos. Poland for decades was a holding and processing center for Russian-mined asbestos. An untold number of workers in the small Polish towns, where asbestos cement factories roared with life during much of the Communist years, are now dying quietly of mesothelioma and other asbestos diseases— even though Russia continues to insist the deaths aren't happening.

In the town of Szczecin, Poland, women used asbestos to knit clothing for their children, and piles of asbestos were stored for years in open containers around the town. In a chilling exposé of the events in Szczecin published by *USA Today* in 1999, reporter Dennis Cauchon revealed the Russian cover-up. "In the Soviet era, asbestos-related deaths essentially did not occur—according to official reports. Studies showing otherwise were censored or confined to a small circle of experts. Even today, some Russian scientists maintain that asbestos-related disease is virtually nonexistent in their country. 'It's a funny thing about Russian asbestos,' said Richard Lemen, a former U.S. assistant surgeon general. 'It causes no health problems at all until it crosses the border, when suddenly and mysteriously it causes cancer.'"

Today, Szczecin has the highest cancer rate in Poland and one of the highest asbestos disease rates in the world. Despite those numbers, Russia continues to be the world's largest asbestos producer, and Russian scientists continue to insist that asbestos diseases rarely occur. Due to Russia's widespread mining, milling, and use of asbestos, it is not only possible, but likely, that an epidemic of asbestos diseases of untold proportions is already taking place inside Russian borders.

SOUTH AFRICA: The legacy of asbestos in South Africa is as grim as in any part of the world. Crocidolite was a major product for years, and workers at the mines had little or no protection. More than 134 mines operated for nearly fifty years, generating profits for the European and South African companies that ran them and enormously high rates of asbestos disease among the workers. Most of the dustier jobs were given to black workers. Until the full extent of the dangers were known, the mines were considered by many to be an ideal place to work because families were able to labor together for the same company. While the men toiled in the mines, their wives often crushed the rock with hammers, separating the raw fibers from the other rock material. The older children usually worked alongside their mothers, while the younger ones played in the debris piles. The result is a nation rife with asbestos victims. A study done in 2001 by Professor Tony Davies from the National Centre for Occupational Health found that more than 95 percent of the women who worked at the mines now suffer from asbestos-related diseases. Many of the mine areas are still highly toxic, as are the estimated four hundred asbestos dumpsites across the country.

JAPAN: Japan has traditionally been one of the highest users of asbestos per capita, importing 220 million pounds of asbestos in 1999 alone, most of it used in asbestos-cement building products. It wasn't until 2000, however, that the country's first asbestos-related death statistics were publicly reported when the Japanese Health and Welfare Ministry released findings that from 1994 to 1998, 2,243 people died of asbestos-caused cancer nationwide. The high number shocked officials, especially given that it included only death certificates that officially listed asbestos as a cause of death. It did not include deaths from asbestosis. The findings, however, were shocking enough to help spur initial plans to ban chrysotile asbestos. Amphiboles have been banned in Japan since 1995. The country is now attempting to develop procedures for identifying, maintaining, and removing asbestos from homes and commercial buildings.

MOROCCO: Like most developing nations, Morocco does not recognize asbestos-related illnesses as occupational diseases despite the fact that the country imports about eleven million pounds of asbestos every year—one-eighth of Africa's annual total consumption, according to the country's Industrial Department. Asbestos use is totally unregulated within the country. Health care and worker protection laws are minimal. The Inter Press Service English News Wire, however, recently reported that medical studies from the United States and elsewhere pointing out the dangers of asbestos are beginning to prompt some debate within the medical and political communities regarding the need for increased worker and consumer safety.

ISRAEL: Crocidolite and chrysotile were used heavily in asbestos cement and water and sewage pipe products manufactured in the city of Naharihya. Workers in the asbestos plant there began suffering from cancer at twice the rate of the national population as early as 1967. Many Israeli homes contain these building products, and abatement is now a concern.

CHINA: A tragedy in the making, China is consuming asbestos at a higher rate than ever before, and observers say the country has no plans to curb its use anytime soon. The Chinese government has made the urgent development of its infrastructure an overriding priority. In the past, China exported a significant portion of the asbestos it mined, but domestic use has increased so rapidly that it now imports asbestos from Canada and other countries. Chinese officials are reluctant to release data regarding asbestos-related diseases

in the country. One of the only sources of information about asbestos in China has been Dr. Liu Shijie, honorary dean at the school
of public health of Beijing Medical University. Dr. Liu told reporters
with the English News Wire that large quantities of asbestos are
being used in building products, cement pipes, and automobile
brakes. In addition, large numbers of Chinese peasants use asbestos
to make stoves and to whitewash their houses. Dr. Liu said that natural veins of asbestos were made accessible to villagers due to the
government's policy of clear-cutting forest lands. In many rural
areas of China, it remains a tradition for new brides to be given
basins full of asbestos so they can whitewash the kitchens of their
homes.

One of the largest asbestos mines in China was long worked by
convicts, many of them political prisoners. The mine, on the frigid
Tibetan plateau, is called Shimian, the Chinese term for "stone
cotton," the local name for asbestos. Historically, China produced
about 25 percent of its asbestos from criminal labor camps.

No medical statistics involving the Shimian workers have been
published, but the nearby villages, inhabited by some 120,000
people, were continually subjected to wind-blown fibers from the
open pit mine, and it was common for middle-aged and older residents to die of "lead lung." Chinese writer Jung Chung wrote about
the "zombie-like" people she saw during a 1969 bus ride past the
prison mine, according to the *USA Today* report. "The faces of the
workers were ashen, the color of lead, and devoid of any animation,"
Jung wrote in her top-selling memoir, *Wild Swans*. Workers in asbestos mines and manufacturing plants in Libby, Tyler, and Manville
gave startlingly similar descriptions of their fellow workers. Oxygen-
starved asbestosis victims often gain a grayish pallor and lack energy,
thus becoming "devoid of animation."

As late as 1997, the United States reportedly imported $17.8

million of asbestos products from China, most of it floor tile, even though the United States officially knew in 1992 that convict labor was being used at the Shimian mine.

TURKEY, NEW CALEDONIA, NORTHERN CALIFORNIA: These three divergent areas of the world have one thing in common— exposure to naturally occurring outcroppings of asbestos. In Turkey and New Caledonia, an island in the South Pacific, communities that exist near the outcroppings of amphiboles have long suffered enormously high rates of asbestos diseases, especially mesothelioma. In both areas, villagers used the asbestos to whitewash their homes. In New Caledonia, the mixture of tremolite asbestos and water is called "Po," and it has been particularly devastating to women, who most often contact the fibers. In Turkey, an amphibole known as eri-onite (which is not officially labeled as *asbestos* by the U.S. government) has proven especially deadly. More than half of the people who die in two exposed villages in Turkey die of mesothelioma.

In El Dorado Hills, California, an elite community about twenty miles east of Sacramento, significant development is taking place in an area laden with serpentine (chrysotile asbestos) and braided with natural tremolite amphibole clusters, similar to those found in Turkey and Libby. Continued development in the area could jeopardize large numbers of workers and residents. EPA studies in northern California have shown that children walking near serpentine-covered roadways over a nine-year period may suffer increased cancer rates of up to 100 times higher than in the normal population. Further studies have shown that tremolite from the foothill region in California is among the most deadly in the world.

These natural exposures, when disturbed either by villagers digging it out by hand to be used as whitewash or by huge bulldozers readying the ground for development, are clearly hazardous, as the stunningly high death rates in Turkey attest.

IRAN, KUWAIT, THE PHILIPPINES, LEBANON, MEXICO, ALGERIA, KAZAKHSTAN, NIGERIA: These are just a few of the developing countries around the world where sources indicate that asbestos workers are often exposed on a daily basis. Dust is present in almost all phases of the manufacturing and handling of the asbestos products, and little or no protective gear is supplied.

There are few countries in the world where a journalist must search far to find an asbestos victim with a grim story to tell. These stories are often gripping and emotional. They convey the worldwide horrors of asbestos in a way that talking about the number of pounds and metric tons being delivered around the globe just can't match.

One such story belongs to Deidre vanGerven, a fifty-eight-year-old resident of New Zealand. Deidre met Thom vanGerven when she was nineteen years old and thought he was the most dashing young man she had ever seen. They were married a year later. Thom, a Dutch immigrant, gained permanent residency in New Zealand and found a job as a bricklayer, rebuilding some of the country's gas works. No one told him the bricks he was handling daily were filled with crocidolite asbestos. He was never given a respirator or any type of protective gear.

In 1989, when Thom was fifty-two, he began suffering a series of ailments, from flus he couldn't shake to frequent pneumonia. He had constant pain in his upper side, and during the night he struggled to breathe. The problems gradually worsened, and the right side of his heart began to deteriorate. In 1997, he had a successful double-bypass surgery.

"He was so excited after the surgery he began planning a trip to Australia to see all his brothers and sisters, whom he hadn't seen in years," said Deidre. "He hadn't been that enthusiastic about life for a long time. It was wonderful to see him like that. Just before we left, he went in for a routine health checkup and they did a lung X ray. That's when they found all the scarring."

She remembers Thom on the way home from the physician's office, saying that he hoped he didn't have asbestosis, which they had described to him as being a long-term, progressive disease. "It turns out he didn't have asbestosis after all," Deidre said. "He had mesothelioma. They said there was nothing they could do. They virtually told him to go home and die."

Devastated by the news, Thom went to bed and closed the blinds. He never allowed them to be opened again. "He suffered terribly after that," Deidre said. "One specialist just shook his head and suggested that Thom take an overdose of drugs. He had fluid drained from his lungs every week. By the fourth week, there were hives all around the hole where the drain was put in. They looked like hives anyway. But they were cancers. If you touched one, he would be in agony. Those same things were all over in the lining of his lungs. Every time he breathed in, his lungs scraped across them, causing excruciating pain. My children were horrified by the way their father died."

Thom passed away in 1997. Time has done little to ease Deidre's loss. She remains frustrated and angry. In New Zealand, as in most countries worldwide, there is no way to sue the companies responsible for exposing their workers. The New Zealand government, too, is immune from any type of legal action.

"There is evil in people who know they are giving workers a death sentence—one in which you spend the last of your days in relentless pain," she said. "They have murdered millions of people around the world and there isn't anything you can do about it. I am not famous, so nobody will pay attention to me. The news reporters here in New Zealand say, 'Oh, that's an old story,' and won't write about it. It's so frustrating. I used to cry every night."

Using the Internet and her telephone, Deidre has attempted to put together a network of people around the globe, many of whom have contacted her to find out exactly how they are going to die. "So many have mesothelioma, and it makes me frustrated that there isn't much I can do. I have no money, and not many governments are interested in helping to find a treatment, let alone a cure."

She lives with the knowledge that she was also heavily exposed because she washed her husband's dusty work clothes for years. "I miss Thom's beautiful face every day," she said. "He should have been able to watch his grandchildren grow up. I wish I could tell the world what a terrible killer asbestos is."

15

BANKRUPTCIES AND
THE COWARDLY LION

O nce plaintiff investigators uncovered the sordid truth—that the asbestos companies knew for decades their employees were getting sick and dying from the fibers—juries across America began finding them guilty in case after case of "failure to warn." As a result, companies began settling the vast majority of cases, and asbestos claims grew into the largest area of product liability litigation in American history.

It might seem that this would be the final chapter in the asbestos story, a Hollywood ending where unscrupulous companies that showed such a blatant disregard for the safety of their workers and consumers would finally pay the price for their actions. But there is a reason that this is not the final chapter.

The legal story of asbestos, far from ending in resolution, has exploded into one of the largest financial and moral dilemmas ever to face American businesses—and the U.S. Congress. The onslaught of asbestos claims has caused more than fifty major U.S. companies to file for Chapter 11, and dozens more may soon follow. Predictions are that more than one thousand American companies may ultimately face asbestos-related legal claims. Cases against the major carmakers in America rose to about thirty-five hundred per month

in 2001 due to the asbestos brakes, gaskets, and other friction parts
that were sold in new cars until recently. The absurdity of the entire asbestos story is perfectly crystallized in the fact that while there
are more than twenty thousand asbestos-related claims pending
against the carmakers, many replacement brakes, marketed mostly
by small, independent brake manufacturers, are still made with
asbestos.

The reason so many companies are being targeted is that after
the majority of the asbestos companies filed for Chapter 11, plaintiff attorneys began looking for other potentially responsible parties.
These included retailers that sold asbestos products, as well as companies that bought or merged with others that had marketed asbestos products in the past. Mainstream American companies like
Dow Chemical Company, Viacom, Halliburton Company, Georgia-
Pacific Corporation, Pfizer, and 3M are all targets that have been
stung by asbestos lawsuits. Estimates are that as many as half of the
major industrial companies in America may face financial challenges
due to the growing number of filings.

At the same time, due to a series of complex legal maneuvers
coupled with questionable court decisions handed down during the
precedent-setting bankruptcy proceedings of Johns-Manville, many
companies—through Chapter 11—are being allowed to severely
limit the amount they are forced to pay to asbestos victims. They are
also effectively eliminating new lawsuits, which was one of their primary goals. To many, this debacle is a final and bitter blow delivered
by governmental and judicial systems that have failed asbestos victims at every turn.

The legal and financial morass first began to form during the first
two decades following WWII, when the asbestos industry, despite
warnings from various insurers, believed it could weather the

handful of asbestos suits and compensation claims that were being filed. The plan worked until the discovery of the Simpson letters and the other smoking guns.

By the 1980s, asbestos litigation had become a "mature tort," meaning that the majority of the evidence against the asbestos companies had already been established in prior trials. It was so clearly and inexorably damning that the asbestos companies saw their futures coming to an end. The mosaic of corporate guilt proven in prior litigation and depositions was so complete that it often resulted in multimillion-dollar verdicts by angry juries in favor of asbestos-cancer victims. The bill for the short-term profits taken by these companies at the expense of the health of their employees and customers was finally coming due, and it was a whopper. By the end of 2001, U.S. companies had paid out more than $22 billion in asbestos claims and related costs. The amount seems high until it is balanced against the costs to the asbestos victims: their health, and often their lives.

For many asbestos victims, including those dying of mesothelioma and other cancers, the jury verdicts were the only vindication they were going to receive. No asbestos company has ever publicly acknowledged its role in poisoning its workers, and no company owner or manager has been prosecuted under state or federal criminal statutes. By winning in civil court, the victims at least felt they were striking the guilty corporate executives in the very place that mattered to them most—the bottom line.

But the Johns-Manville bankruptcy proceeding, which took years to complete—during which time asbestos victims were not paid a penny—changed all of that. It remains one of the most important and underreported financial news events of the latter part of the twentieth century. It is a story that brims with enough plot twists, legal machinations, and human moral dilemmas to easily fill a book on its own. The outcome was critical because it remains the

basic model for many of today's Chapter 11 filings involving asbestos claims.

In the end, after tens of millions of dollars were spent on legal
and experts' fees and the issue had been dragged through the courts
for more than a dozen years, the "bottom line" looked like this:
While Johns-Manville paid its debts to commercial creditors on a
dollar-for-dollar basis and was allowed to do business as usual, future asbestos claimants were paid ten cents for every dollar they had
won from the company through the legal system. That lasted until
July 2001, when the amount dropped to five cents on the dollar. As
a result, most mesothelioma victims, who often face up to a half-
million dollars in health care costs to help them battle the enormous
discomfort of the incurable disease, were regularly paid less than
$20,000 by the J-M Trust.

"It's a complete travesty of justice," said Scott Handler, a Texas
plaintiff attorney, who echoed the sentiments of hundreds of thousands of asbestos victims nationwide. "Johns-Manville got away
with mass murder. These companies were dirty; they took risks with
people's lives. There is a reason why all these juries keep finding
them guilty. These bankruptcy laws negate the plaintiff's right to a
jury and create a blueprint for taking corporate America off the
hook for conduct that has devastated people's lives."

In 1982, when Johns-Manville ran for cover under the blanket of
Chapter 11, it controlled an estimated 25 to 40 percent of the national asbestos product market. The company was more than sol-
vent; it was robust, with revenues of $2.2 billion. It was ranked 181st
on the Fortune 500 list. The company had plenty of cash to pay off
liabilities due to more than sixteen thousand lawsuits already filed
against it by asbestos victims. It greatly feared that future claims
might skyrocket, however, and its concerns were underscored by

warnings from insurance companies, which were posturing themselves to limit their own liabilities. By the early 1980s, about five
hundred cases a month were being filed by asbestos claimants. Most
were settled out of court, but what really frightened J-M executives
was the fact that they were losing more than half of the cases they
took to court, many of which had large punitive damages attached.
In one lawsuit alone, a jury awarded retired boilermaker James
Cavett, who was dying from asbestosis and lung cancer, a total of
$4.8 million.

In August 1982, Johns-Manville shocked the corporate world
by becoming the first financially healthy American company ever to
seek Chapter 11 protection. The company's argument was that it
needed time to reorganize—not because it was insolvent, but because it feared it might become insolvent in the future.

Asbestos claimant attorneys filed an extensive motion to have
the Chapter 11 filing dismissed, complaining that the maneuver was
simply a ploy by the company to delay payment of their asbestos liability while figuring out a way to avoid future liability. The court,
however, denied the motion and allowed the unique proceeding to
continue.

For the next four years, the J-M bankruptcy slogged through
the mazelike proceedings of Chapter 11. The company filed reorganization plans, which were batted around and took several years
before being approved. No asbestos claims were paid during the interim. Meanwhile, the company was doing a brisk business domes-
tically and overseas. For example, for the third quarter of 1988—the
year the reorganization plan was finally approved and the company
was discharged from bankruptcy court—the company had a net income of more than $53 million on sales of $584 million. It is not
known how many asbestos victims died of their diseases during this
time. Those statistics, unlike the company's monthly profit and loss
statements, were not kept.

During those six years, the company was allowed to do business as usual, despite the fact that juries across the country had
found that J-M had intentionally exposed its workers to asbestos and
in fact owed those workers tens of millions of dollars. Some argued
this was necessary because to shut down the company and sell off its
assets to pay for the asbestos claims would have deprived future
claimants a chance to collect on their claims. Others argued that,
from a moral standpoint, Johns-Manville should have been forced
into a final bankruptcy, with every last paper clip sold off to pay the
asbestos victims' claims.

In 1988, the bankruptcy court in the Johns-Manville case put its
faith in a little-tested procedure whereby two trusts—a Personal Injury Trust and a Property Damage Settlement Trust—were created
as sources of payment to the asbestos claimants. The trusts were to
be independent entities from the company. They were funded
largely through a combination of cash, accrued interest, insurance
settlements, and, initially, 50 percent of Johns-Manville's common
stock. A percentage of the company's annual profits were also scheduled to go to future claimants.

The trust plan may well have worked more efficiently for both
sides had it not been for two things. First, despite the fact that the PI
Trust soon had an executive director and more than ninety employees, it was poorly administered, according to a judicial review
of the trusts in 1990.

Far worse was the fact that by 1989, the PI Trust had announced that it was running out of money. The PI Trust had been
grossly underfunded. J-M was ordered back into bankruptcy court
in 1990 to increase funding and restructure the operation of the PI
Trust. Ultimately, the trust received 30 percent more of the J-M
stock for a total of 80 percent. During this time, asbestos victims

who were owed money by the company lost out again as another freeze was put on payments by the court. It took five years before the freeze was lifted. Inexplicably, the PI Trust was once again greatly underfunded. By the time the PI Trust was back in business in 1995, it had already received nearly three times more claims than the court had anticipated for the lifetime of the trust.

Barred from returning to the company for more funds by a court order, the PI Trust, in 1995, paid asbestos claimants ten cents and then, finally, five cents on the dollar. Meanwhile, the company continued to pay its regular vendors the full amount it owed them for goods and services. The company was now safely distanced from the asbestos claimants, and it quickly prospered once again. Recently, Berkshire Hathaway purchased J-M, including all of the J-M stock, for more than $1 billion. The current Johns Manville Company—now without the hyphen—has ten thousand employees in fifty-five locations around the world. Sales last year were at $2 billion.

There are those who argue today that the PI Trust was funded with every excess penny the company made beyond what it needed to survive. They point to the fact that the PI Trust is still worth $2 billion and is at least paying out some money to asbestos claimants. Others say the entire deal was a sham. What is known is that the structure and funding of the trusts were the responsibility of the court, which relied on an agreement negotiated primarily among company attorneys, asbestos claimant attorneys, and a court-appointed attorney who was supposed to represent the rights and interests of the future asbestos claimants.

Many of the asbestos claimant attorneys involved in the deal today argue that there was no way of predicting the skyrocketing number of plaintiffs who would file against J-M after 1995. They were, like the court itself, caught flat-footed with surprise. Even if they had predicted the number correctly, they argued, there simply wasn't enough money in the company to pay the staggering number of asbestos claims on a dollar-per-dollar basis.

Yet the fact remains that in the deal approved by the court—and which served as a blueprint for other Chapter 11 filings—the commercial creditors received 100 percent of what was owed to them, the existing asbestos claimants received most of their claims, the courts got rid of a frustrating and embarrassing situation they hadn't been able to solve in more than a decade, and the future asbestos claimants' representative was well compensated and rewarded by the court for his work in expediting the process. *The only ones left out in the cold in the deal were the hundreds of thousands of future claimants, many of whom were just beginning to get sick.* The ruling, among other things, barred them from having their day in court. They were no longer allowed to face and accuse the company that had poisoned them or to seek damage awards that might actually pay for the huge medical bills many of them faced down the road. At the same time, the company had gotten what it wanted most—the elimination of future jury awards and a minimal payout required on all future claims.

One observer wryly noted that before 1800, bankruptcy laws called for a guilty defendant to be flogged while his ear was nailed to a post. "In this case," he said, "justice might have been better served."

In the 1990s, dozens of companies that had sold asbestos products saw the J-M Chapter 11 as a way out from under the crush of legal claims being filed against them. At the same time, some of the asbestos companies began dismantling their corporate structure by spinning off various subsidiaries and divisions prior to filing for Chapter 11.

It was this process that W. R. Grace began to follow as it became more evident in the late 1990s that asbestos-related claims against the company were only going to increase. It had weathered the out-of-court settlement with the families of the eight leukemia victims in Woburn, Massachusetts, and even its portion of the nearly $70 million cleanup fee it paid the federal government for the massive pollution it left at the Woburn site.

But on April 2, 2001, the company filed for protection under Chapter 11, announcing that the asbestos claims were too huge for the company to handle. At the time, Grace had annual sales of about $1.6 billion and more than six thousand employees worldwide. The company reported it had settled more than fifty-three thousand asbestos claims for a total of $1.25 billion and was a defendant in more than sixty-one thousand pending cases. The number was growing daily against Grace, having increased by 81 percent in 2000 alone.

In a press release, Grace officials said the company would work closely with asbestos claimants to develop a reorganization plan that would "address valid asbestos claims in a fair and consistent manner and establish a sound capital structure for long-term growth and profitability."

The filing infuriated the asbestos victims in Libby. "It's a slap in the face," said Gayla Benefield. "They promised to pay the medical expenses of the people whom they poisoned up here, and now this is their first move to void that promise and to get out from under the debts they owe. It's a sham and a disgrace."

While the other companies have waltzed through their Chapter 11 proceedings and were awarded vastly reduced payments to asbestos claimants without much fanfare, the Grace bankruptcy attempt ran smack into a the stubborn forms of Paul Peronard, the EPA, and the U.S. Department of Justice. Fearing that Grace will try to avoid paying for the cleanup in Libby, the EPA joined what could be a precedent-setting lawsuit against Grace. The agency joined asbestos claimants in charging that Grace fraudulently shifted billions of dollars in assets out of the company in the 1990s to shelter the funds from the asbestos claims and the cleanup charges. The EPA alleged that the reorganization of the company was simply an illegal effort to gut the original corporate core, leaving only a shell to go through the bankruptcy. Named in the suit were companies that assumed the businesses spun off by Grace, most notably the Sealed Air Corporation, a leading worldwide manufacturer of packaging materials located in Saddle Brook, New Jersey.

Asbestos plaintiff attorneys who filed the suit charged that the complicated Grace reorganization was not an attempt to "address valid asbestos claims in a fair and consistent manner," as the company claimed, but a maneuver to hide and protect its profitable businesses from the onslaught of asbestos claims.

The EPA charged that the company drained off assets and funds that should have gone to clean up not only Libby but also scores of other sites around the United States polluted by Grace. The lawsuit sought to unwind the spin-off transactions, returning perhaps more than $5 billion to Grace's creditors. The Sealed Air Corporation and the other defendants denied all charges and vowed to defend their interests "vigorously."

The outcome of the legal actions will have huge ramifications for dozens of other companies contemplating Chapter 11 to avoid escalating asbestos claims. It is the asbestos story's gunfight at the OK Corral, with billions of dollars at stake.

With hundreds of thousands of lawsuits already pending, the financial threat of the asbestos litigation to American business is a serious one, and it appears far from over. The stakes are monumentally high and the issues complex and volatile. Without exaggeration, there is nothing less at stake than the future of dozens of American corporations and the quality of health care for tens of thousands of asbestos victims. It is an issue that deserves far more attention from investigative news reporters around the country.

Unfortunately, what has captured the imagination of much of the media has not been the stories of the victims, the culpability of the industry, or the controversies inherent in the Chapter 11 process. Rather, it has been the spectacular nature of the *projected* financial numbers associated with the growing number of lawsuits. The Rand Corporation, among others, published predictions that the number of asbestos lawsuits against American companies may reach as high as 1.5 million in the near future. Headlines in the nation's top business publications—many of which are owned by huge corporations now involved in asbestos litigation—have screamed for the past few years that the total cost of asbestos litigation may reach $200 billion. Typically, they neglect to include the fact that the reason for this is the asbestos industry knowingly exposed more than one hundred million Americans— and the number rises daily—to a substance the industry knew was highly toxic. Rarely is the number of preventable asbestos-related deaths among American workers and consumers included in these articles.

Nevertheless, the fact is that asbestos litigation remains an ominous storm cloud hovering over the futures of hundreds of companies. It is an issue that has left the companies, lawyers on both sides, and the media scrambling to assess blame. It has also left Congress on the sideline, unable or unwilling to craft a solution to the problem. The list of companies that have already filed for protection under Chapter 11 include the following:

A.P. Green 2002

Harbison-Walker

    Refractory Co. 2002

Kaiser Aluminum 2002

North American

    Refractory 2002

Eastco Industrial Safety

    Corporation 2001

Federal Mogul 2001

G-I Holdings

    (formerly GAF) 2001

Skinner Engine Company ..2001

USG Corp. and subsidiary

    U.S. Gypsum 2001

U.S. Mineral 2001

Washington Group

    International 2001

W. R. Grace 2001

Armstrong World

    Industries 2000

Babcock & Wilcox 2000

Burns & Row Enterprises ...2000

Owens Corning 2000

E. J. Bartells 2000

Joy Technologies 1999

Rutland Fire Clay 1999

Atlas Corporation 1998

Brunswick Fabrications ...1998

Fuller-Austin Insulation ...1998

M. H. Detrick 1998

SGL Carbon 1998

Rock Wool Manufacturing 1996

Lykes Brothers Steamship ..1995

American Shipbuilding ...1993

Baldwin Ehret Hill 1993

Keene Corp. 1993

Cassiar Mines 1992

Kentile Floors 1992

Eagle-Picher Industries ...1991

H.K. Porter Co. 1991

Celotex

    (Philip Carey Co.) 1990

National Gypsum 1990

Standard Asbestos Manufac-

    turing & Insulation 1990

Delaware Insulations 1989

Hillsborough Holdings ...1989

Raytech (formerly

    Raybestos-Manhattan) ..1989

Waterman Steamship

    Corp................1988

Gatke Corp. 1987

Nicolet 1987

Todd Shipyards 1987

Pacor 1986

Prudential Lines 1986

Standard Insulations Inc. ..1986

United States Lines 1986

Forty-Eight Insulations ...1985

Wallace and Gale 1984

Amatex 1982

Johns-Manville 1982

At first glance, the list is startling, including American business icons like Kaiser Aluminum, Babcock & Wilcox, and Owens Corning. The reaction for many people reading such a list for the first time is a visceral one—what is this thing eating away at the very core of the American business structure? Without a full knowledge of what precipitated these actions—which includes the information that has convinced hundreds of juries across the country to find the executives of these companies guilty of egregious deception and disregard for human life—the reaction of most Americans is anger aimed at the asbestos victims and their attorneys. The asbestos industry, including those companies now being threatened, has taken full advantage of that reaction. It created a new promotable villain, one that is perhaps the easiest to sell to the American public this side of big tobacco—plaintiff lawyers.

In a flood of articles, press releases, and public statements, corporations facing asbestos claims have blamed "greedy" plaintiff lawyers as the reason these lawsuits exist in the first place. They claim plaintiff lawyers represent people who are often not sick and that excessive lawsuits have clogged up the courts and threaten America's very way of doing business. The asbestos victims themselves are rarely criticized because sick people don't usually make effective promotable villains. The plaintiff attorneys, though, are an entirely different matter.

One of the more grievous charges frequently made against the plaintiff attorneys pursuing asbestos-related cases is that they are paralyzing America's court system through the sheer number of filings. It is a concept that seems to have taken root despite the fact that, according to the Association of Trial Lawyers of America, an average of fewer than seventy asbestos-related lawsuits actually go to trial annually in state and federal courts—hardly a paralyzing number.

The real controversy over these filings centers on the fact that some plaintiff lawyers have conducted a mass screening of potential victims and have produced huge numbers of claims on their behalf. In some mass claims, victims who suffer from cancer or advanced asbestosis are combined with others who may suffer from pleural thickening or who simply have been exposed to fibers. The strategy enrages defense attorneys, who claim it is a form of legal blackmail. Many argue that claimants who suffer only from "markers," which are plaques and other lung scars caused by the fibers, are not truly sick and should not be included with cancer victims.

The situation raises two critical moral and financial issues. Within the first issue, two questions have to be asked. Should companies that had nothing to do with poisoning workers be liable for damages? And if not, who should pay for the terrible suffering of the victims?

These are difficult questions to find unbiased answers to because everyone involved has a stake in the outcome. The defense, of course, would like to make this first question the only issue, ignoring the guilt of the asbestos industry and the enormous pain and sickness of the people it victimized. Plaintiff lawyers, who have the law on their side, believe it is justifiable and necessary to follow the corporate chain to the core companies even if they were not directly responsible or negligent. One such case involves the Texas-based Halliburton Company, which faces hundreds of thousands of asbestos-related claims, most of them inherited from Dresser Industries, a company Halliburton acquired in 1998 while under the management of U.S. Vice President Dick Cheney. Cheney served as chairman and chief executive of Halliburton from 1995 to 2000. He engineered the $7.7 billion acquisition of Dresser Industries, believing that the escalation of asbestos-related claims against that company had almost run its course and that Halliburton's insurance would shield it from the costs of future legal claims. Like other chief executives at the time, he was badly mistaken. When Cheney left the company in August 2000, Halliburton's stock sold for more than $54 a share. In September 2002, after the number of asbestos claims against the company had exploded, it had dropped to below $15 a share.

CBS, a company that never sold or marketed asbestos products, is also facing asbestos claims because the broadcasting company, in 1968, purchased Lorillard, a company that manufactured Kent cigarettes. In the early to mid-1950s, the company put crocidolite asbestos into the "micronite" filters of more than twelve billion Kent cigarettes. CBS purchased the company long after the asbestos was taken out of the filters.

Viacom, which owns CBS, is also weathering a storm of asbestos-related claims that it inherited due to its 2001 purchase of the Westinghouse Electric Company. Westinghouse used asbestos in its appliances and has been hit by more than 130,000 lawsuits, according to the *Chicago Sun-Times*.

The second issue is equally critical. Defense advocates argue that American companies are being victimized primarily by people who aren't really sick. A group of plaintiff lawyers who represent only mesothelioma and other cancer victims are also calling for victims who are not sick to be eliminated from the ranks of claimants. That would leave far more funds available for their clients, whose medical needs are immediate and whose diseases are often incurable. The law, however, allows advocates for all of those exposed to file claims, and that is what plaintiff attorneys are continuing to do. Although most Chapter 11 companies are paying only pennies on the dollar on asbestos claims, many claimants are able to collect from multiple defendants. The total amount they receive, however, is still usually nowhere near what it would be if their cases were tried before a jury.

One concern of those who have been exposed to asbestos is that if they do not proceed with their legal claims, they will lose their standing due to the variety of state and federal statutes of limitations. Moreover, plaintiff attorneys are well aware of the flight of so many companies toward Chapter 11. They fear that if they do not file claims quickly, the companies may not be available as defendants in the future.

The key issue, however, is medical, not legal. Some defense advocates have argued that those with pleural abnormalities are not really sick, even though many of them may ultimately lose a significant percentage of their lung function. If the findings of Dr. Alan Whitehouse and others who have dealt extensively with asbestos victims are correct, and pleural disease is progressive and can be fatal, then the defense should rest on that issue.

The missing entity in all this has been the U.S. Congress. This is a billion-dollar issue involving the future of scores of American companies and hundreds of thousands of American workers who have been exposed to a toxin that the U.S. government failed—and continues to fail—to regulate properly. Yet Congress has done nothing to help resolve any of these dilemmas. Most of the past legislative efforts heavily favored the industry and were quickly defeated through opposition by trial lawyers and the unions. Most of these bills involved tax breaks and bailouts for the industry and severely restricted the victims' rights and abilities to seek compensation from the companies involved.

Although most observers are doubtful that it will happen, it is clearly time for Congress, like the cowardly lion, to find its courage and tackle the problem. To do so, however, means that it must find a way to resist the enormous pressures of industry because its first priority must be to find ways to provide medical care for the victims of asbestos-related diseases. It should also investigate the Chapter 11 procedures used by companies hoping to escape the barrage of asbestos claims. Currently, there is no meaningful oversight of the process, nor any evaluation procedure to determine whether it is working in a fair and equitable manner. Part of that evaluation should include a possible redefinition of Chapter 11 laws so that guilty corporations cannot escape paying the cleanup costs of the sites they have contaminated.

Perhaps the stunning paradox of our asbestos policies can be best seen in the fact that although the mining, manufacturing, and commercial use of the fiber has led to catastrophic health problems for hundreds of thousands of Americans and bankruptcy for dozens of major companies, and while U.S. workers and companies have lost hundreds of billions of dollars because of it, and will continue to do so into the foreseeable future, asbestos remains a legal ingredient in thousands of American products.

16

COVER-UP
AT GROUND ZERO?

Without question, one of the strangest and most frightening twists in the asbestos story took place in lower Manhattan in New York City in the eight months following the destruction of the World Trade Center. Boiled down to the essentials, scientists are saying that the EPA and other government officials literally overlooked—perhaps intentionally—the asbestos fallout around Ground Zero. It is a deadly serious accusation because if it is true, thousands of visitors and residents of lower Manhattan may have needlessly been exposed to potentially lethal fiber levels. The result could be tragic. For those exposed to the underdetected asbestos levels in lower Manhattan after September 11, the increased cancer rate could go as high as one in every ten of the most heavily exposed people, according to Cate Jenkins, a scientist with twenty-two years of experience in the EPA's hazardous waste division. As has been the case in the story of asbestos from the beginning, this should never have happened.

It was strange enough that the North Tower of the WTC had a direct tie to Libby. Monokote, the fireproofing spray made by

W. R. Grace, had been used in at least the bottom thirty-nine floors—and perhaps as high as the seventy-ninth floor—of the North Tower. Even more bizarre, however, were the reactions, following the terrorist attack, of governmental agencies, including Region 2 of the EPA, which has jurisdiction over Manhattan. Their baffling actions lent credence to the haunting idea that asbestos somehow corrupts or confuses those in power who come in contact with it. It is at least one explanation for the shocking and inexplicable fact that in the hours and days following the collapse of the WTC, the EPA knowingly allowed outdated dust sample analysis equipment to be used—equipment that failed to detect the true levels of asbestos in the dust spread from the WTC throughout the surrounding area. Even more curious is why Region 2 officials turned down a free loan offer of not only far more efficient analysis equipment—equipment that would ultimately reveal dangerously high levels of asbestos in areas of lower Manhattan—but also a team of some of the most highly trained asbestos field investigators in the country.

One of the few places in Manhattan where the more efficient dust analysis equipment was used was Region 2's own building at 290 Broadway, according to Jenkins. Excessive levels of asbestos fibers—which were not detected with the equipment that was used by the EPA to study dusts in most of the rest of Manhattan—were found and, even as New Yorkers were assured it was safe to return to their homes and businesses, the EPA closed its building for nearly a week to clean the asbestos contamination. The agency did not advise anyone else in the city to take similar measures.

Adding to the bizarre nature of the events surrounding the search for asbestos is the fact that a highly reputable private testing firm found high levels of asbestos near Ground Zero shortly after the WTC collapse. Yet their findings were mysteriously removed from the Internet shortly after they were posted and the firm was told that its services were no longer required.

In the days following the September 11 attack, as Wall Street reopened and people returned to their homes upon being reassured that the dust cloud that had enveloped the area was essentially harmless, Region 2 EPA field investigators, for reasons still unknown but to a few, used polarized light microscopy (PLM) to sample for asbestos fibers in the dust and soils. This occurred despite the fact that the PLM technology is outdated and could not detect most of the thin asbestos fibers in the WTC dusts. According to Jenkins, the proper test method should have been the use of transmission electron microscopy (TEM), which is far more sensitive and can easily detect even asbestos fibers pulverized by the 1.2 million tons of debris from the WTC.

The difference between the TEM and PLM instruments is years of evolutionary technology. Whereas a TEM instrument can detect asbestos fiber levels as low as 0.0001 percent, PLM can reliably detect only 1 percent or higher levels of asbestos.

Jenkins said TEM is the current prescribed methodology in EPA guidelines for studying asbestos in dusts and other solid materials whenever PLM cannot detect it. TEM is also required for air monitoring, and the EPA did use it for that purpose in Manhattan. However, it was not used to analyze the asbestos content of the dust, even though TEM has been used in most other asbestos investigations, including the EPA's sampling of soils in Libby, in a large asbestos abatement project overseen by Region 2 in Manhattan in 1998, and for dust in the first bombing of the WTC in 1993.

EPA officials in other areas have tried to reason why Region 2 didn't order the use of the TEM method to analyze the dust by explaining that other health entities, including those from New York

State and New York City departments, as well as outsourced private firms, were responsible for much of the early sampling efforts and did not have access to, or chose not to use, the TEM instruments.

This explanation raises two questions. First, why didn't the EPA, which has far more experience and expertise, take control of the asbestos sampling? The second question is far more troubling. Within hours of the collapse of the WTC, Region 8 officials in Denver, Colorado, offered the New York investigators the use of some forty TEM and scanning electron microscopy (SEM) instruments. The SEM instruments are similar to TEM in their superior ability to detect the microscopic fibers. These were accessible because the Denver office had contracted them for use in Libby. The offer included a dozen of the more modern microscopy instruments that could have been rushed into lower Manhattan within twenty minutes by car. At the same time, the Denver office offered to immediately send some of the Libby asbestos strike force—dozens of highly trained and experienced field investigators who were experts at collecting and analyzing asbestos samples—to help gather data in Manhattan. This was a team that had already taken hundreds of litigation-quality air data collections in Libby. The question that has yet to be answered is why the entire offer—from the more modern microscopy to the strike force team—was turned down by Region 2 officials.

Meanwhile, although environmental tests from at least one private firm using TEM instruments showed disturbingly high levels of asbestos, the green light was given by the EPA to the people of lower Manhattan to return to their homes and businesses.

This seeming contradiction was exposed by sources inside the EPA and in an explosive memorandum written by Jenkins. In a memo originally released on March 11, 2002, with data added on April 30 and May 7, Jenkins outlined the litany of mistakes made by Region 2 in the aftermath of the WTC collapse. Her allegations were stunning. In a cryptic heading of the memo, she summarized:

EPA Region 2 knew TEM was required and needed, had it after the WTC collapse for their building, used it in past, but refused to use it for the rest of NYC.

She blasted Region 2 for not abiding by the EPA's own requirements that asbestos dusts be analyzed by TEM, and then dropped a bombshell by accusing EPA officials of deliberately concealing the fact that they had used the more sensitive equipment on their own building.

Region 2 had positive TEM results, but negative PLM results on the exact same dust samples, for its own building after the WTC collapse, and abated for asbestos based on these TEM results. They were apparently sensitive after this fact. Region 2 failed to supply the relevant TEM dust and other data for their own building in response to a FOIA (Freedom of Information Act) request. Region 2 also obscured the fact that TEM dust testing was performed on its building as part of a February 22, 2002 letter from EPA Administrator Whitman to Congressman Jerrold Nadler (D-New York). In an attachment to that letter, Region 2 indicated that only PLM testing was performed.

Although EPA officials continually assured New Yorkers they faced no asbestos contamination after the WTC collapse, sampling data showed otherwise. Soil and dust samples taken in an apartment on Warren Street, four blocks from Ground Zero, and analyzed with TEM, showed 79,000 fibers per square centimeter of asbestos. "These are levels worse than many of those in Libby before the cleanup," Jenkins said. "In general, in terms of quality of testing, there is a difference of night and day between the ways they tested in New York versus how they are testing in Libby."

Jenkins's memo included a table that compared TEM and PLM

results taken at two sites, one at 150 Franklin Street and the other at 200 Rector Place. At the Franklin Street site, nine dust samples were taken from places such as the roof, elevator shaft, and windowsills. The PLM tests found that only two of these samples showed slightly elevated fiber counts. The TEM tests showed highly elevated and dangerous fiber counts in every sample. At the Rector Place address, none of the PLM tests turned up detectable fibers, while the TEM tests found fibers at every location. Similarly, at the EPA Region 2 building on Broadway, PLM tests showed no fibers in five samples that included dust from the lobby and outside the building, while the TEM tests again found fibers at every location. Jenkins also noted that EPA investigators in Libby found "high levels" of fibers in area soils using TEM and SEM, while no fibers were detected using PLM.

At least one private, independent sampling firm also found elevated levels of asbestos almost everywhere it sampled. The Virginia-based H. P. Environmental testing firm analyzed dust from two buildings near the WTC site and found that seven of eleven samples they analyzed exceeded the EPA's threshold level for asbestos. The fibers were at first hard to detect because they were shattered. It wasn't until the company's scientists, Piotr Chmielinski and Hugh Granger, used TEM that they found the telltale fibers. Their report stated: "The data suggest a greater potential for worker exposure to asbestos within building structures than previously reported for outdoor rescue and recovery work in the area around the World Trade Center." The report also warned that because most of the asbestos fibers were even smaller than normal, they were especially dangerous. "Within building structures, it should be anticipated that very small asbestos fibers may become airborne and remain in the breathing zone of workers for extended periods."

But the story of Chmielinski and Granger doesn't end there. Anxious to share the information with the scientific community, the two professionals posted their findings on the Web site of the American Industrial Hygiene Association. Within hours, the asbestos report was removed from the site, with no explanation to either man as to why. Less than twenty-four hours later, Chmielinski and Granger were notified that they had been taken off the job and they were no longer needed at Ground Zero. Just who intervened and sabotaged the work of H. P. Environmental—and why—remains a mystery.

Region 2's decision not to use the TEM generated a withering storm of criticism. CNN quoted Hugh Kaufman, former chief investigator for the EPA's Ombudsman Office, as saying, "I believe EPA did not do that because they knew it would come up not safe and so they are involved in providing knowingly false information to the public about safety. Not just EPA. . . . All the agencies, local, state, and federal, have been consorting together every week to discuss these issues."

Kaufman went so far as to say that Whitman's statement that the air in Manhattan was safe was "false." He called the contaminants, especially the asbestos, a substantial health hazard. Kaufman, who was removed from his position by Whitman last year, and has since filed an action under the whistleblower protection provisions, has long been at odds with Whitman over the level of the EPA's cleanup of some Superfund sites.

Representative Nadler also ripped into the EPA. He called the EPA's air quality green light "erroneous" and called into question the "integrity" of the agency's testing methods. He also held hearings that questioned directives to Manhattan residents that the asbestos in their homes and apartments could be eliminated by using a wet mop or wet rag.

Jenkins also criticized Region 2's claim that the asbestos concentration in WTC dusts was low and not a health hazard. She wrote in her memorandum, "This directly contradicts the findings of the extensive risk assessment for Libby where the same concentrations, occurring less frequently, were the basis for placing Libby on the Superfund list. . . . Dusts from the collapse of the WTC present more risk than soils in Libby because they are finely divided surface dust with no vegetation to hold them in place."

Some EPA scientists have countered Jenkins's argument with the theory that risk assessments cannot be made based on the asbestos content of dust or soils—only by the fiber levels in the air. Investigators in Libby, however, found that both sets of information are critical. Their conclusions were that if there are fibers in dust or soils within human traffic areas—such as in carpets or on sidewalks or playgrounds—sooner or later the fibers will be disturbed and become airborne.

Further criticism was leveled at the EPA because the agency refused to monitor the interior of buildings, homes, and apartments before giving the "all clear" for residents to return to their homes and businesses. Although the EPA took on the job of testing the outdoor areas around the WTC, it delegated the task of testing interior environments to New York City agencies. The city, in turn, passed that job on to building owners, landlords, and residents. As a result, few indoor tests for asbestos and other toxins were done, yet people were repeatedly told by local and federal health agencies that these environments were safe.

During the turmoil, Jenkins illuminated an issue that at first glance may seem little more than a bureaucratic argument, but is, in fact, a critical oversight. Throughout the days and months following the WTC terrorist attack, the EPA, NIOSH, and OSHA continually referred to asbestos in the WTC dust as being either above or below the 1-percent mark. All three agencies assumed the 1-percent level as the "safe" benchmark for the amount of asbestos found in dust samples.

"That's an absolutely false and potentially dangerous assumption," charged Jenkins. "You have to be very careful dealing with the agencies in New York; they will definitely try to convince you that you don't have to worry about asbestos levels below 1 percent and it simply isn't true."

The problem is that the 1-percent threshold does not apply to dust levels but rather to the EPA's definition of asbestos-containing building materials, according to Jenkins. Moreover, the 1-percent threshold was never based on health issues and was never meant as a "safety" level. It was established at a time when only PLM existed and there was no way for investigators to reliably determine the number of asbestos fibers under 1 percent. According to Jenkins, the 1-percent threshold was created due to the limitation of the microscopy equipment, not its threat to human health. Studies show that soils or dust containing 0.001 percent asbestos can be unsafe. This is especially disturbing considering that the "1 percent" rule was exceeded by more than one-third of the samples of bulk dust taken near Ground Zero during the first week after the attack.

"EPA REGULATIONS AND GUIDANCE STATE THAT 1% IS NOT A SAFE LEVEL," Jenkins's memo concluded in capital letters. "In a January 25, 2002, speech, Counsel for Region 2, Walter Mugdan, also stated that the 1% level was not a health standard, but only the detection limit of the PLM method," she wrote.

Region 2 still wasn't finished making critical mistakes, according to Jenkins. While soil sampling can tell investigators how much asbestos is likely to become airborne when disturbed, air samples themselves are vital in understanding the immediate dangers. Region 2 investigators claimed on the EPA Web site and elsewhere that the air standard set by the Asbestos Hazard Emergency Re-

sponse Act (AHERA) is "70 structures per square millimeter."
Jenkins said that once again Region 2 used the wrong standard. In
her report, Jenkins wrote:

- "Region 2 falsely claims 70 structures/square millimeter is
  AHERA standard."
- "The actual AHERA standard for asbestos in air is ZERO."
- "There is no other EPA ambient air standard other than
  ZERO asbestos."

She also stated that the air standard level labeled as "safe" by
Region 2 is actually four to eight times higher than asbestos air contamination levels found inside residences in Libby.

The question that begs an answer is why the secrecy and deception
in New York? Why did Region 2 turn down the use of the TEM instruments and the skilled asbestos field investigators? And why were
the combined governmental agencies in such a hurry to assure
people they were in no danger when, in fact, the potential for asbestos exposure remained high?

It would be logical to assume that out of a fear of financial
panic in the nation following the September 11 attacks, the White
House felt it was a top priority to get Wall Street up and running as
quickly as possible. It also may have been a priority to cloak the total
damage done by the terrorist attack to hide the true vulnerability of
America's cities.

Another possibility is that given the administration's close ties
to corporate America—and the fact that thousands of U.S. companies are currently being sued over asbestos claims—it may have
hoped to downplay the dangers of asbestos.

Bureaucratic ego or an unwillingness to step on other agencies'
toes may have played a part in terms of why Region 2 officials turned

down the offer for the TEM/SEM instrumentation and the investigators; or they may have truly, if mistakenly, believed that they and the other governmental agencies involved could handle the problem themselves. Much of the earliest sampling done was conducted by teams from Con Edison, which has always used PLM to investigate possible asbestos contamination from breaks and explosions in their network of steam pipes in Manhattan, according to Jenkins.

It could also be that the proper analysis methodology fell through the cracks as bureaucratic buck-passing sent responsibility for indoor asbestos sampling from the EPA to city officials and finally to local landlords. For now, it is all speculation, but the people of New York deserve answers to what remains a potentially deadly mystery.

Much has been written about the Monokote that was sprayed onto the North Tower. The manufacturer, W. R. Grace, advertised the product for years as being "asbestos-free" although it contained tremolite and the other amphiboles from the mine in Libby. Grace continued to sell Monokote until 1973, when the federal government banned the spraying of asbestos fireproofing. (The ban was inexplicably overturned in the early 1990s, according to EPA officials.)

However, the majority of the asbestos found in the WTC dusts was chrysotile. The findings underscore the fact that most buildings in New York, like every other major city in the United States, contain high levels of the "white" asbestos. For example, the H. P. Environmental report stated that the WTC towers contained up to 8.5 million square feet of vinyl chrysotile asbestos floor tile. It was also used on the structural steel, in the elevator shafts, on decorative finishes in the lobbies, and possibly in the drywall and foundation concrete.

The exact amount of asbestos in the WTC towers and the other buildings that were destroyed in the terrorist attack is not known, but some estimates range as high as one thousand tons. What is known is that those who witnessed the application of the asbestos during the WTC's construction in the late 1960s and early 1970s were often shocked at the level of use.

One witness was Dr. Irving Selikoff, who was appalled at the procedure. In an intraoffice memo, W. R. Grace executives described Dr. Selikoff's reaction as he spoke before a health conference in 1969.

> *[Dr. Selikoff] leveled very serious charges about the definite danger created by the use of sprayed fiber fireproofing. He then turned to sprayed fiber fireproofing in New York, showing the unchecked 'snow' throughout the downtown area. Special note was made of the World Trade Center. Selikoff stated they estimate 100 tons of fiber will be airborne in New York from this job. He closed by stating the work practice was the worst he could imagine and from his observations not one man spraying fiber today would be alive in 20 years. The officials of the international unions were there along with contractors and I know it landed like a bomb.*

The unions' concern helped put a halt to the spraying of Monokote and other fireproofing sprays on the WTC. New York, however, is a city full of asbestos. In a report presented to the National Academy of Sciences, Laurence Molloy, owner of the Molloy Corporation, a New York environmental management firm, stated, "An estimated 68 percent of all buildings in the city are sources of 'invisible' asbestos exposure."

One theory that caught the imagination of some in the media was that if the WTC towers had been filled with asbestos they may not have burned. This rumor enjoyed widespread circulation before it was disavowed as scientifically inaccurate by engineers and researchers who studied the dynamics of the attack. "You could have packed both towers with asbestos all you wanted and it wouldn't have had an effect," said Dr. Thomas Cahill, the University of California at Davis physicist who studied the collapse dynamics. "The fire was far too hot and the floor literally sagged away from the walls as the lateral beams melted and bent. Any statement that more asbestos would have saved those buildings is totally inaccurate."

Of all the revelations that took place in New York following September 11, one that should not be overlooked is the exposure of firefighters and other rescue workers to asbestos. Obviously there were a number of other chemicals in the toxic soup that polluted the air after the WTC collapse, but firefighters are constantly faced with asbestos exposure during their careers. Results of a 1990 study released by the Division of Environmental and Occupational Medicine at Mount Sinai School of Medicine indicated that 20 percent of the chest X rays of 212 participating New York firefighters showed pleural thickening and other abnormalities caused by asbestos exposure. Recent studies of current New York firefighters found similar results.

The problem is not only the initial airborne fibers from the fires, but the dust that collects on uniforms, equipment, and even on the fire trucks. Exposure often occurs after the fire is out and firefighters take off their masks only to inhale fibers shaken off their clothes or equipment. Asbestos is also often used inside the firehouses and in the firefighters' gloves, coats, and boots to fireproof them.

Clearly, local and federal agencies should make it a priority to develop ways to protect firefighters and rescue workers from this deadly exposure. The men and women who put their lives on the line to help others should not have to face additional dangers they can't even see.

Under pressure from a number of sources, the EPA announced in May of 2002 that it would help fund and conduct the cleanup and testing of apartments and residences in lower Manhattan. The *New York Times* called the move a "sharp reversal in policy by the EPA," which had said all along that indoor spaces were not its responsibility. Under the plan, the EPA, New York State, FEMA, OSHA, and other local agencies agreed to collaborate on the cleanup—done by certified contractors—and follow-up testing for asbestos in the apartments of residents living south of Canal, Allen, and Pike Streets. The cleanup, which began in September 2002 and could include up to fifteen thousand apartments, was a welcome move, but many believe it should have been done months earlier.

"It is a shame that these measures were not taken at a time when they could have prevented the heavy exposure to the toxic dust that covered lower Manhattan," said Joel Shufro, executive director of the New York Committee for Occupational Safety and Health (NYCOSH), a coalition of unions and health professionals. "For nearly eight months the EPA has denied that it has authority to protect people from exposure to toxic substances indoors. Now the EPA is taking responsibility for protecting lower Manhattan residents, an action which it could have taken months ago."

Despite their "reversal of policy," the EPA did not move from its public stance that little health danger was presented by the asbestos from the WTC. It continued to stand by its statements that most of the air samples taken were below "levels of concern." Jane Kenny, the EPA's Region 2 administrator, told reporters that the cleanup process "is not an emergency. What we are doing now should ensure that there is no potential for long-term health risk." There was no official reaction to Jenkins's allegations that the "safety levels" the EPA used were highly inflated. Whitman also never addressed her often-repeated statement that it requires long and lengthy exposures to asbestos fibers to cause disease—a statement that has been proven false in Libby and elsewhere.

As the cleanup of lower Manhattan continues, the questions surrounding the EPA Region 2's handling of the asbestos dangers from the WTC remain unanswered. The pressure to find out why the agency acted as it did will likely diminish over time because, as has happened so often in the past, the long latency period of asbestos diseases will dull any clear and immediate consequences regarding the decisions that were made. It will be ten to twenty years and perhaps even longer before the final page of this chapter can be written.

17

THE $500 MILLION
SILVER BULLET

*"A friend of mine read about all this in the paper and told
me he was afraid he had been poisoned too. He described his
symptoms; they were the same ones I have. He had full-
blown asbestosis and didn't know it. He's dead now. This
isn't going away. We need help up here."*

—*Bob Dedrick*

In Montana, winter is the familiar season. For most of the residents
of Libby, the long cold is a solace, a rest from the riotous energy of
spring and summer. To Paul Peronard and the troublemakers of
Libby, though, the winter of 2001 was anything but peaceful. The
enormity of the human tragedy in northwestern Montana was hitting
home. Nearly fourteen hundred people were being treated for asbestos
diseases, and more than two hundred had already died. In some cases
entire families had been struck down. Harvey Nobel worked at the
vermiculite mine for thirty-one years before he died of advanced asbestosis in 1990. His wife, Dorthe, died of asbestosis in November of
2001, and all eight of their children were diagnosed with asbestos-

related diseases. The family now fears for the grandchildren, who are not yet old enough for symptoms to have shown themselves.

Despite the plague of death and sorrow that had been unleashed on the community, it seemed to Peronard that W. R. Grace opposed every move the EPA made to clean up the town. Their obstructive actions and uncaring attitude infuriated him.

"They lied to us, interfered with us, and have never acknowledged what they did here to the people of Libby," Peronard said. "Grace is the most evil company I've ever dealt with. They are Satan in corporate clothes."

As the number of stricken residents grew, the health care costs in Libby skyrocketed to an estimated range of from $500 million to $1.5 billion. They dwarf the yearly budget for St. John's Lutheran Hospital in Libby, which averages about $15 million. Peronard and the health care officials in Libby feared that although some of the cost would be borne by health insurers, it was possible that treating the asbestos victims could financially overwhelm not only the hospital but also the city, Lincoln County, and perhaps even the state. Grace was the logical place to look for financial help, but the company's Chapter 11 filing greatly complicated the issue. The multibillion-dollar corporation had promised many times that it would always be there for the sick people in Libby. But if the core of Grace dissolved during bankruptcy, Libby residents feared that its promises would dissolve as well. In the bitterest of ironies, those who had been poisoned by the mine operation now had to hope the company responsible remained financially healthy and profitable. Sometimes it felt as though all reason and justice had fled from Libby. In the early winter of 2001, not much made sense anymore.

For Peronard and the EPA team, the battle with Grace had become trench warfare. Grace attorneys bickered with the EPA over every

THE $500 MILLION SILVER BULLET   295

detail, including the agency's method of sampling and analyzing asbestos within the homes of Libby. Initially, the company fought to
have the lesser-powered PLM instruments used to count fibers
rather than the newer and more powerful TEM. As *The Spokesman-
Review* in Spokane pointed out in an editorial, "This is the same
company that used new technical information to claim it did not
pollute the water in Woburn, Mass. . . . It seems new technology was
fine when it was beneficial to the company's position but is not
when it may show higher levels of asbestos."

(Grace CEO Paul Norris in 1998 denied that the company was
responsible for the leukemia deaths in Woburn. In a letter to Grace
employees and retirees, he wrote: "I've taken a very close look at
Grace's actions leading up to, during and since the Woburn trial and
I am confident that we did not contaminate the drinking water in
Woburn.")

The EPA ultimately won the battle to use the TEM and SEM
instruments in Libby, but Peronard and the EPA team were deeply
angered by Grace's recalcitrant and arrogant attitude. The company
was habitually slow in turning over documents and information and
fought the EPA over the technical details of the cleanup process. In
the spring of 2002 it also began turning down about two-thirds of
the people who applied to the medical program the company had
set up for asbestos victims in Libby. Until that time it had accepted
nearly every applicant into the program. Some of the people the
company began excluding were workers who had spent more than
a decade in the mine at the dirtiest jobs, according to Dr. Brad Black.
One man, upon returning home after extensive surgery was performed on his lung due to an asbestos-caused condition, found a
letter from Grace stating that he did not warrant qualification in
their medical program.

"I've never dealt with a more uncooperative, irresponsible, interfering, unconscionable company in my career," assessed Peronard.

"I can't describe how bad it has been working with these people. The last thing they are thinking about is trying to help the families in Libby."

Even the company's occasional press releases infuriated the EPA team and the Libby troublemakers. After Grace promised to donate a quarter of a million dollars a year "for as long as necessary" to the hospital to provide independent health screening, company representatives added: "We take our responsibilities to the people of Libby and the situation there very seriously. This is a unique situation deserving a dedicated solution. People who have concerns about possible exposure to asbestos now will have an independent place to go and be tested. If anyone is diagnosed with an asbestos-related illness, they will have insurance to cover the medical costs of treating it."

The EPA team could only shake their heads at the wording. *If anyone is diagnosed?* How could anyone in good conscience write something like that, Peronard wondered.

The company concluded its statement by pledging: "We stand by our commitment to do the right thing for the people of Libby. We will continue to be responsible to the people of Libby affected with asbestos-related diseases."

Grace's Chapter 11 filing left many people wondering whether the company would uphold any of its promises. In a letter to Governor Judy Martz, Montana's attorney general, Mike McGrath, warned that the growing cleanup costs in Libby would likely be borne by the state and the EPA. "It is my opinion that Grace will not legally be able to perform a voluntary cleanup," he wrote in August 2001. "The bankruptcy process will preclude Grace from spending money in Libby."

McGrath urged Martz to encourage the EPA to include Libby

as a federal Superfund site on the National Priorities List. Martz, sensitive to the concerns of the Libby business community, which continued to fear the stigma of a Superfund designation, remained cool to the idea.

The Grace Chapter 11 filings had a depressing effect through-out Libby. It seemed clear that Grace was distancing itself from the town. Certainly the Chapter 11 filing had thrown into limbo the one hundred pending asbestos claims and the hundreds and perhaps thousands of future claims against Grace by Libby-area asbestos vic-tims. After viewing the precedent set by the Johns-Manville bank-ruptcy, the claimants feared their opportunity to seek financial justice from Grace had just vanished.

The local newspapers reported that under existing federal laws, the average Libby asbestos victim could receive as little as $400 from Grace. Although lawyers, lawsuits, and litigation were foreign and generally distasteful concepts to most Libby residents, they never-theless knew that asbestos-related diseases were expensive to treat. The fact that Grace appeared to be on its way toward legally shed-ding financial responsibility for cleaning up the asbestos pollution and for the medical care of poisoned residents left many people de-pressed and angry.

It didn't help that Grace was still a highly profitable and thriving company whose executive officers received annual multi-million-dollar packages that included salaries, bonuses, and stock options. Given that kind of available money, $250,000 per year for medical care for an entire town seemed a ridiculously small amount.

As the Montana winter closed in, Libby was in need of some good news. The troublemakers—Benefield, Skramstad, Wilkins, Dedrick, Racicot—and others like Mike Switzer; Neil Bauer, the outspoken

town barber who could give you a haircut for eight dollars and debate Grace's tactics at the same time and who, along with his twin
brother, was diagnosed with asbestosis; and Clinton Maynard, who
also has asbestos scarring and whose father, a sweeper in the dry
mill, was killed by asbestos poisoning in 1989, continued to attend
the Citizen Advisory Group meetings and voice their opinions, but
progress was exasperatingly slow. Still, they made up a vital part of
the force created by a disparate group of Montanans who just years
before had never heard of words like "amphibole" and "mesothelioma," and who had never written to a public official in their lives.
Yet by the winter of 2001, they were among the world's most edu-
cated people on the dangers of tremolite exposure. Even as the
media began pulling back on the story—Libby is off the beaten path,
after all—the troublemakers stayed active. They wrote letters, made
phone calls, combed through endless and hopelessly complicated
medical and financial reports, and struggled their way through the
various governmental bureaucracies, most of which still believed
that asbestos is a problem of the past. While Grace had highly paid
lawyers and world-renowned consultants, Libby had housewives,
barbers, carpenters, and retired miners dying of asbestosis. As motivated as the troublemakers were, in the winter of 2001, it didn't
seem like a fair fight.

Elaborate landscaping in Libby has always been perceived as super-
fluous. Nature laid such a spectacular hand to the mountains and
forests ringing the town that lush lawns and well-clipped hedges
always seemed a bit self-important and insignificant by comparison.
Besides, extensive landscaping requires the kind of discretionary
income that is not readily available in Libby. One of the few properties in town with a perpetual fresh coat of paint and manicured

grounds is the funeral home near Mineral Avenue. Business has been good there lately.

Montanans are a self-sufficient people, though, and most residents of Libby treasure their gardens. Most of the modest homes lining the wide, flat streets are surrounded by small, sparse lawns, but in the corners nearly all of them sport verdant, healthy gardens. Since the 1950s, Libby residents believed that the secret to their bountiful yields of fruit and vegetables was the soil amendment they received at discount rates—and sometimes free—from Grace. The gold, puffy vermiculite was a perfect soil additive. Porous and water absorbent, it was a natural soil aerator and moisturizer. Most of the gardens and lawns planted before the mine closed in 1990 were full of Edward Alley's magic mineral. When the snows melted back into the earth in the spring, the garden plots often glistened gold in the sun. Most people in Libby saw it as a harbinger of another good crop year, until they learned the truth.

For Peronard and the EPA, removing the vermiculite from the hundreds of gardens and lawns in Libby was the beginning of a challenge so large that no one in the agency had ever faced anything like it. The EPA had cleaned up a dozen or two homes in a site before, but never an entire town. In fact, the cleanup at Libby was the largest project any U.S. agency had ever encountered. The cost was projected to be nearly $100 million, and the source of funding remained unclear. Various options were discussed and debated in the Citizen Advisory Group meetings and within the EPA. Most felt Grace should pay the entire cost, but getting more money from the Chapter 11–protected corporation was going to be difficult.

As the winter set in, there was only one thing for certain: Removing the deadly vermiculite was going to transform the lawns

and gardens in Libby into the most expensive landscaping in
America.

Throughout the summer and fall of 2001, the most contentious option for cleaning up the town was the Superfund designation. The
business community, particularly the real estate agents and others
who relied heavily on clients from outside Lincoln County, remained vehemently opposed to the Superfund. Who would want to
buy a house or property in a town that was officially declared a polluted disaster area? The troublemakers, on the other hand, were convinced that it was the only way to get the town cleaned up. Grace
certainly wasn't going to voluntarily pay for it. The company still
hadn't admitted it had done anything wrong. It seemed to Benefield,
Skramstad, Wilkins, and the others that the only viable financial option left was the Superfund.

Congress established the Superfund Program in 1980 as a ve-
hicle to clean up the thousands of uncontrolled and abandoned
hazardous waste sites created primarily by manufacturing and processing plants throughout the United States. The key element of the
program is the Superfund Trust Fund, which receives most of its
money from taxes on chemical and petroleum industries. It is used
primarily when the companies or individuals responsible for the
contamination cannot be found or forced to pay for the cleanup
work. Embedded in the program is the "silver bullet" option given
to the governor of each state. By using the silver bullet, a governor
can designate any specific site within the state to immediately be
placed in the Superfund program. The "speed" element of the silver
bullet was crucial because a key dilemma facing Libby was the
lengthy delay usually inherent in the Superfund designation
process. Hundreds of residents—including children and infants—

were being exposed daily to the tremolite fibers in their homes, lawns, and gardens. The silver bullet would speed up the cleanup process by more than a year. The only problem was that each state gets only one silver bullet request, and Montana had other highly polluted mining areas. Still, it was hard to imagine a town more in need than Libby.

Clinton Maynard, who had originally struck upon the idea of using the silver bullet when he found that Montana was one of only seven states left that hadn't yet used their silver bullet, led a letter-writing campaign to Governor Martz, while Skramstad and others made personal pleas to her. The soft-spoken, gentlemanly Skramstad had met Martz before, and the two had struck up a friendship. Although his lungs were steadily shutting down because of the asbestosis—he struggled for breath even on short walks—he and Norita made the 350-mile trip to visit the governor in Helena.

Despite his personal feelings toward Martz, Skramstad knew convincing her wouldn't be an easy task. Despite her grandmotherly looks and warm smile, she was a tough, savvy politician. She had run on the slogan that Montana was "Open for Business" and considered most environmentalists as obstructionists. She created the Office of Economic Opportunity in 2001 specifically to stimulate business in Montana. Convincing her to side against the Libby business community wasn't going to be easy.

Martz, however, was well aware that the issues in Libby had gathered nationwide press. In August she made a well-publicized trip to Libby for a town meeting and a tour of the area. She listened intently as Peronard, in his rapid-fire fashion, laid out the scenario, including the dangers that still existed for many Libby home owners. Yet she remained noncommittal. "Don't assume I'm leaning one way or another," Martz warned the emotional crowd at the meeting, most of whom were pleading for her to utilize the silver bullet.

Martz's appearance in Libby was followed by a visit by the EPA's Whitman, who pledged support for the community. Whitman carefully described the Superfund as a potential option for a house-to-house cleanup. Peronard, as he had done so many times before, had already gone out on a limb for the people in Libby and recommended that the town be included on the National Priorities List as a Superfund site. His position did not please some business owners, but Peronard believed it would ultimately benefit them as well. The nation already knew that Libby had been contaminated; the only solution seemed to make it clear to everyone that it was being cleaned up.

The *Montanian* newspaper supported the Superfund designation but pointed out that even if the majority of the local residents of Libby asked for the designation, the governor and state environmental officials could effectively torpedo the request.

In October, Martz dropped a bombshell by announcing she had decided against the use of the silver bullet in Libby. It was a crushing blow to those who had lobbied for the Superfund.

"We were terrified that if we didn't get something to happen, the EPA would just leave town and we would be stuck with hundreds of homes that were still contaminated," said Skramstad. "That would have exposed an entirely new generation of children to the asbestos fibers. We were getting desperate."

As the weeks went by and the cold fronts pushed down out of Canada, a solution seemed more elusive than ever. It seemed ironic that the very insulation that kept many of the homes warm in Libby was more deadly than the freezing temperatures of winter. A gloom settled over the town, but when the change came, it came suddenly. On the afternoon of December 20, 2001, the Citizen Advisory Group members and others in Libby were surprised to be invited to a hastily called meeting at the Libby Town Hall. Martz had arrived and was going to make an announcement. Nobody seemed to know what it was all about. Dedrick and Racicot were there, wondering what the governor was going to say. Dedrick felt it had to be something positive for Libby, otherwise why would Martz make such a special effort? He even felt she might be there to announce something about the Superfund designation, but everyone around him disagreed. After all, Martz had been adamant about her opposition to it.

Racicot wasn't sure what the governor was up to, but he knew the Libby activists had put her in a tough position. They had applied pressure in every way they knew how—including the stories in the national press—and he hoped the pressure was enough to make her do something to help the town.

About fifty other residents showed up, each wondering what they were going to hear from the governor. Many were angry and ready to confront her about her reluctance to include Libby in the Superfund. They were restless and still shuffling around for seats when Martz took the podium. Without preamble, she said: "I am announcing my decision to support a Superfund decision for Libby. But I am truly not here just to announce the designation. I am here to announce to you that I will utilize Montana's one and only silver bullet."

Although Martz couldn't suppress a smile as she made the announcement, it took a long moment for the news to sink in to the stunned audience. Then, scattered applause began to build and finally the crowd rose to its feet. Racicot was shocked. A friend sitting beside him—an ex-military officer Racicot had known since childhood who was now dying of asbestos-related cancer—had tears in his eyes. Racicot knew his friend was terrified that his family was also going to fall victim to the fibers. "I didn't think she was going to do it," the man said, his voice breaking. "I just didn't think she was going to do it."

Dedrick joined heartily in the standing ovation. Although he had predicted good news, he could still barely believe what he had just heard. Finally, an answer seemed within grasp. The cleanup would take years to complete, but at least the town now had a chance.

Martz didn't elaborate on the reasons behind her change of heart. She told the audience only that she had rejected the silver bullet option in October because in the aftermath of the September 11 attacks she feared a potential terrorist strike that could cause an environmental disaster worse than the one in Libby. Some residents believe that at least some of the business community had finally come to believe as Peronard did—that the town's future rested with the Superfund designation.

In the end, most of the people in Libby didn't care why the governor had changed her mind, only that she had. The next day, a local paper ran a picture of Martz making her surprise announcement. The huge headline above the photo read: "Merry Christmas."

For the Libby activists, the governor's announcement was the culmination of years of fighting against long odds. "It really picked us up," said Racicot. "There is an old saying that 'you can't fight city hall' but you can, by God, take a backhoe to it, and that's what we were ready to do. The governor's agreement to use the silver bullet came just in time because things seemed pretty grim. It gave us some hope."

Martz's use of the silver bullet also prohibited opponents of the listing from stopping or delaying the process. Grace never indicated it would contest the designation, but most residents were comforted by the fact the company was seemingly prevented from interfering.

While buoyed by the fact that they had been given the green light to clean up the town, the EPA teams knew it wasn't going to be easy. They were faced with the daunting task of stripping out the vermiculite from more than a thousand homes. In August 2002, the EPA's HazMat teams began cleaning the first house in Libby.

Peronard remained the focal point of the operation. The trust that he had engendered within the community remained the most critical component to the project. He was still working fifteen-hour days, handling the thousands of questions and logistical challenges the cleanup project generated, and preparing for hours of depositions as a precursor to the bankruptcy lawsuit against Grace. His ulcer wasn't getting any better.

The logistical problems faced by the cleanup teams were extraordinary. What was planned in Libby had never been done before in the United States—not at Love Canal, Woburn, or any of the thousands of other contaminated sites across the country. Perhaps only the Wittenoom story in Australia was comparable. In Wittenoom, however, the town was simply abandoned, its residents moved by the government to another site. "The truth is, it would have been more cost effective to do the same in Libby," said Dan Thornton, the EPA environmental scientist who had tried to track the vermiculite trail nationwide. "Given the housing costs in northwestern Montana, it would have been less expensive to demolish the town and cap and contain it than clean it up. Obviously, we would have run into some substantial resistance with that option. We can't just go in there and tell people they have to move, but it probably would have made economic sense."

Bob Wilkins agreed that few people would have gone along with a relocation plan. "I know it would probably be cheaper to do that," he said with a small grin, "but money sure isn't the reason we all live here. I've been here a long time. I know it will never be the same place it was before we found out what Grace did. But, at some point in your life, you have to dig in and defend your ground. This is my home."

Racicot agreed. "The small-town magnet is powerful. The town gets inside you. A lot of people here haven't been any farther than Spokane. They don't want to be worldly. But I guess this time the world came to us. Should we have been ready for it? I don't know. If you look at what happened in other places, including New York after September 11, I think you'll see they weren't ready, either. The point is, nobody should have to be ready for what happened here."

For the troublemakers of Libby, the past three years haven't been easy ones. They have all been diagnosed with serious asbestos-related diseases, as have numerous friends and family members. The odds of them winning their battles against Grace—as well as against the rest of the town—were never good. But without them, the tragedy in northwestern Montana may never have been exposed. Maybe they didn't knock down city hall with a backhoe like Racicot envisioned, but there is no question they finally have the government's undivided attention. After sixty years, the asbestos poisoning of Libby is coming to an end. Unfortunately, due to the latency period, at least one more generation will suffer before the final death toll can be figured.

For Dedrick, the situation in Libby continues to be a matter of fighting one battle at a time. A large part of his ability to manage his anger—which reappears every morning as he watches his wife,

Carrie, struggle with the physical manifestations of advancing asbestosis—is to take a measure of satisfaction with each small victory.
"The goals we set in the beginning were the cleanup and the medical screening," he said. "We're a bunch of small-town people with
no experience in this kind of stuff, but we achieved both of those
things. Now, what is really needed is long-term medical funding. We
also have sick people here who need help. We need money for them
right now. I'm focused on that."

For Skramstad, justice won't be fully served until those who
knew about the asbestos dangers and failed to tell the workers so
they could protect their families are criminally prosecuted. "If they
ever try any of them for criminal charges, I don't care if they hold
the trial in Afghanistan, I'll be there," he said. "I believe that the top
people at Grace, who made those decisions, should be on trial for
their lives—just like we are."

For Benefield, the Superfund designation was bittersweet. It
marked an amazing accomplishment—one she could never have envisioned in the desperate days following her mother's death.
Without Benefield's stubborn will and substantial resolve, the full
story of Grace and the vermiculite mine may have never emerged.
With Grace struggling legally and financially, Benefield has done her
part in keeping her promise to her mother, a promise that had motivated her during the difficult times when it seemed as though no
one wanted to listen to the truth. Yet even though her struggle has
finally been vindicated by most of the town, she knows that any satisfaction she feels is diluted by the fact that so many of her friends
and family are suffering from asbestos-caused diseases.

"This town and I have been through enormous changes," she
said. "It wasn't that long ago that I really didn't think there was a
chance to expose what Grace did to this community," she said. "I
was just so angry at what they had done to my mother and father, I
had to keep trying. In the next two years, I went through it all—

from being nothing but trouble in the community's eyes, to being called in the middle of the night by people I barely knew who asked me things like, 'What do I do? I was just told that I am dying.' It is hard to feel like you've won when you hear that. I could have walked away from the town, but my children and grandchildren live here. They can't leave. I have a responsibility. We all do."

Throughout the summer of 2002, Benefield helped the Citizen Advisory Group play a key role in the EPA cleanup and its efforts to find funding sources for the escalating medical needs of the community. She was also contemplating a run for public office. "I don't want what happened to us to happen ever again—anywhere," she said. "But it is clear to me now that if we are going to change things, we have to do it ourselves."

For his work in Libby, Peronard was named the EPA's National On-Site Coordinator of the Year. He was honored in a formal ceremony in Washington, D.C., by Whitman, who presented the award. It marked one of the first times his friends had ever seen him out of his trademark blue jeans and T-shirt. Peronard, who had hoped his work in Libby would be finished by Thanksgiving back in 1999, now estimates that the house-to-house cleanup won't be completed until 2006. "It's Stalingrad," he said.

The experience has left an indelible mark. "You don't ever get to nirvana on this job," he said. "It's all about damage control. There are too many people who have lost their lives or who have lost a family member to ever claim victory. Even if we are successful in all our legal endeavors, they are all about cash. We'll get some money for medical care and that's a good thing, but it isn't full satisfaction—it isn't justice. That will never be found here. But I know we are making progress in Libby, and that's worth fighting for."

18

TOWARD BANNING
ASBESTOS

In the summer of 2002, U.S. Senator Patty Murray of Washington introduced a bill to do something that should have been done long ago—ban the use of asbestos in the United States. A domestic ban on asbestos is the first of a number of actions that must be taken to stop the health and financial plagues that asbestos has perpetrated on America and the world. A ban is critical because Americans are unknowingly being subjected to exposure every day. Testifying before Congress in July 2001, Dr. Richard Lemen, former acting director of NIOSH and former assistant surgeon general, said that the number of household products containing asbestos, including washing machines, dishwashers, toasters, furnaces, floors, and ceiling tiles—as well as textile products such as clothing, yarn, thread, cord, and string—is increasing each year. At the same time, millions of pounds of asbestos are being used annually in the construction of new homes and buildings in the United States. Far from being a problem of the past, asbestos is still legal and still killing us.

The regulatory agencies' effort to monitor what Paul Peronard calls the "most important toxin of our time" remains one of the most deadly governmental failures in U.S. history. Anna Knudson, an asbestos expert who helped Senator Murray draft the legislation, said that asbestos is one of the least-controlled substances in America.

"We know American consumers and home owners are being exposed," Knudson said. "It's just frightening to realize that nobody knows to what extent. No agency is tracking asbestos products except in emergencies, and even then most don't even use the right sampling equipment. We asked the agencies if they were updating their asbestos sampling technologies and if they were paying attention to asbestos issues. The overwhelming answer was no to both questions."

Like other regulatory agencies, the EPA does not routinely perform tests on toxic substances, according to the EPA's 2001 Office of Inspector General Report. "Instead," the report concluded, "EPA usually relies on those who make or use a substance to develop adequate data on the substance's effect on human health and the environment." This statement sums up the absurd and impotent approach government regulators take toward asbestos. Not only do regulators rely on an industry that has repeatedly proven to be duplicitous in its actions—including the frequent alteration and omission of critical scientific data—but the various and overlapping state and federal agencies don't agree on sampling methods, technologies, or even asbestos threshold safety levels.

The agencies' response to this is inevitably that they are not funded properly to do the types of monitoring and testing necessary. In part, this is true, and that point must be addressed by the present and future administrations if they are serious about showing the world the United States truly cares. The abysmal failures in Libby by state and federal regulators, however, had nothing to do with budget restraints. These deadly shortcomings were due, in large part, to past regulators serving the wrong master. Future efforts should be patterned after the example set by Peronard, Chris

Weis, Dr. Aubrey Miller, and the rest of the EPA team in Libby. Their efforts, methodology, and courage to speak out and fight to uphold the law should be the model for all government regulators to follow.

Senator Murray's bill—officially, the Ban Asbestos in America Act, Senate Bill 2641—calls for a variety of needed actions, including a phaseout of all importation and distribution of asbestos-containing products by 2005 and a ban of the six regulated forms of asbestos. It would require a nationwide study of the present dangers that products like brake pads and building materials—as well as asbestos-contaminated products like vermiculite—present to consumers and workers. Further, it calls for expanded medical research on asbestos-related diseases and the creation of a National Mesothelioma Registry to improve tracking of the disease. Finally, it would require the EPA to convene a panel of experts to study the adverse health effects of nonasbestiform minerals such as talc and other durable fibers.

The bill is long overdue for there is no ethical, economic, or practical justification for the continued use of asbestos. Only the uniformed or economically involved still argue that asbestos is not a dangerous and often fatal substance. Hundreds of worldwide studies, including those financed by the asbestos industry, have proven that asbestos fibers are harmful and often lethal. No reasonable scientist or physician today argues otherwise. Moreover, other industrialized nations have banned it, finding better alternatives for nearly every use. The question isn't whether America should ban asbestos, but rather why it has taken this long to do it.

One of the greatest tenets of this country is our professed belief in human rights. It is time we put that belief to work here at home. In the United States, an estimated fifty thousand blue-collar workers die each year from illnesses caused by workplace exposure, according to OSHA. That is an astounding number; yet it is largely unreported and ignored. Blue-collar workers remain what Brodeur once scathingly referred to as "expendable Americans." His work remains a seminal voice in protest of the treatment of this segment of society, but it has easily been drowned out by the howling chorus for bigger and faster profits.

Part of the blame must be laid at the feet of the unions and the workers themselves, who are often too willing to overlook poor working conditions in exchange for higher pay during negotiations. But far too often, workers and consumers are not being informed of the dangers they face. The past failures of governmental regulatory agencies are part of it, but the dark heart of the problem is the fact that corporate executives, as evidenced throughout the entire story of asbestos—as well as in today's headlines—often follow their own code of morality, which places financial success above all else.

In the spring and summer of 2002, when it became apparent that there were corporate "irregularities" being conducted within companies like Enron and WorldCom, Congress and the Bush administration were quick to call for new laws that imposed criminal sanctions on the perpetrators. Vice President Cheney told the Commonwealth Club in San Francisco, "Where there is corporate fraud, the American people can be certain that the government will fully investigate and prosecute those responsible."

It is telling that the "corporate fraud" in question involved money, not worker and consumer safety. For generations, the asbestos industry caused the deaths of blue-collar workers and consumers nationwide, yet there was no outcry for corporate justice from anyone but a handful of vocal victims. While it is laudatory that government is today vowing to punish corporate financial wrongdoers, that definition should clearly be extended to those who knowingly manufacture and sell toxic products.

The justice system has not hesitated to prosecute owners of asbestos abatement companies who violate the law by doing their jobs improperly and exposing workers and sometimes area residents to fibers in the process. There are many incidences where people have been sent to jail or prison for improper abatement practices. Few would argue the justice of these prosecutions. Those who knowingly expose others to a deadly toxin should be criminally prosecuted. If that is the case, however, the question must be asked as to why those within the asbestos industry who knowingly exposed workers and consumers haven't been similarly prosecuted.

Banning asbestos in the United States is also critical for the country from a financial standpoint. Asbestos products have a tremendously negative value in the long run. By ignoring and sometimes hiding the need for safety precautions in the workplace, the asbestos industry has cost itself—and the nation—far more than the price of installing proper safety equipment and enforcing stringent workplace safety laws.

"It didn't make any sense," said Peronard. "The asbestos industry conducted a powerful and concerted effort to make us [government regulators] go away. They tried everything they could to maintain the status quo, even though they knew it was harming the lives of hundreds of thousands of people. Then they got the hell sued out of them and many of them ended up filing for Chapter 11.

There was nothing logical about it, unless you figure the only thing they cared about was short-term profits."

The result is the biggest and most bizarre legal tangle in U.S. history. Hundreds of companies may file for Chapter 11 protection due to the hundreds of thousands of workers' claims, yet the vast majority of the workers themselves will be left with little or no recompense. Congress is faced with a Gordian knot that must be severed in such a way that American business is not derailed, while at the same time victims are provided full health care coverage and the opportunity to seek damages for their suffering. Faced with such dire financial consequences, how can lawmakers justify allowing the continued sale of the very products that caused these problems in the first place?

Despite the overwhelming evidence that the Murray Bill is decades overdue—and would undoubtedly save hundreds of thousands of Americans from being exposed to the deadly fibers in the future—the reality is that the bill may well fail when it is considered by Congress sometime in 2003. The asbestos industry is well entrenched and will pull out all stops to try to kill it quickly. Perhaps even more problematic is that bill supporters must overcome the inertia among the vast majority of Congress members, who, like the rest of America, are under the mistaken impression that asbestos has already been banned and is a problem of the past.

Finally, supporters will fight an uphill battle trying to educate colleagues that asbestos is a present and future danger. Senator Mark Dayton of Minnesota, a cosponsor of the bill, said he did not know asbestos products were still legal in America before he talked with Senator Murray. "I didn't realize it hadn't been banned," he told reporters. "It seems so obvious and common sense. Once again corporate greed has triumphed over the greater good in this country."

Even if the Murray bill fails, the effort to ban asbestos must continue until the job is done. Anything less is condemning future generations to a deadly toxin and our own for allowing it to happen.

The United Nations recently stated that asbestos is responsible for one hundred thousand deaths annually worldwide—and that number is expected to increase until the international trade in asbestos is halted. The U.N.'s Interim Chemical Review Committee has recommended restricting the global trade of asbestos. In sanctioning the international trade of asbestos, the United States has consistently sent the wrong message to the rest of the world. In a real sense, we are turning our backs to the inevitable and terrible suffering that will occur among workers and consumers in developing nations for decades to come. It is an unconscionable and indefensible action. To meet our moral duty as the leading industrial power in the world, the U.S. must do more than ban the importation and use of asbestos within the country. It must join the effort to ban asbestos worldwide.

Governments in nearly every other industrialized country in the world have already banned asbestos use. By doing so they have not only reduced the levels of suffering and death for future generations, they have met the ethical and human obligations they have to the people they are pledged to protect. The European Union nations, Australia, Japan, New Zealand—all have recognized the recklessness of supporting the industry. The World Health Organization (WHO) has long called for an international ban on asbestos. "The WHO recognizes what NIOSH concluded twenty-five years ago, in 1976, that . . . only a ban can assure protection against the carcinogenic effects of asbestos," testified Dr. Lemen.

If the international trade in asbestos products is not halted soon, it could produce a hundred-year wave of sickness and death in developing countries. In addition to the immense human suffering involved, continued use of asbestos will, inevitably, lead to economic chaos within these countries as health, legal, and abatement costs skyrocket. And what do these countries receive in return? A short-term earnings boost benefiting a handful of companies and government officials who profit from the trade.

Another critical issue the U.S. government must address is the ongoing exposure to asbestos abatement employees and do-it-yourself home remodelers. Along with mechanics who handle brake pads and asbestos-containing engine parts, they comprise a large portion of what medical experts fear will be the next wave of asbestos-disease victims. With millions of tons of asbestos in buildings and homes in every state, renovations and demolitions can produce extremely high fiber levels in the atmosphere that can endanger the workers, nearby pedestrians or residents, and the future occupants.

A large number of asbestos abatement workers are young males, many of whom are immigrants. Both groups tend to be easily exploited, as young men often tend to think of themselves as invincible and don't bother with proper safety equipment or methodologies if their supervisors don't seemed concerned about the dangers. The problem is greatly compounded by the fact that it is likely that the majority of asbestos abatement projects nationwide take place without any type of permit process, protective equipment, supervision, or monitoring. If this situation does not change, hundreds of thousands of workers and building occupants may suffer high exposure levels in the decades to come.

Federal and state agencies might do well to study the situation in Texas, where a potential solution to at least part of the problem was implemented following a series of investigative reports done by the *Austin American-Statesman*. The newspaper uncovered the fact

that asbestos abatement laws were being ignored in about 90 percent of the renovations and demolitions statewide. This included the
abatement of more than three thousand commercial and governmental structures in central Texas every year, according to reporter
Kevin Carmody. Most state and federal regulators agree that similar
potentially deadly scenarios are being played out across the nation.
In California, for example, a 1988 study by the state legislature
found that more than 70 percent of the asbestos removal work done
in the state was not inspected by a public agency. "Consequently,
there is a high likelihood that much of this unchecked work is not
being done safely," the California Assembly Office of Research report stated. No follow-up to that report has ever been done.

Carmody outlined a potential solution to at least part of the
problem, which should be considered for use nationwide. He found
that the city of San Antonio refused to issue permits for renovation
or demolition of commercial buildings unless the owners had a li-
censed consultant survey for asbestos. The survey had to be completed and presented to the permitting agency, thus making it
harder for an owner to argue ignorance of the law. At the permitting stage, the owner is informed of all the safety procedures that
must accompany an asbestos abatement project. City officials said
more than 95 percent of the owners comply with the survey requirement.

Inspired by the articles in the *Austin American-Statesman*, the
Texas legislature in 2001 passed legislation that required a similar
process statewide, banning the reinstallation of asbestos in public
buildings and tightening rules on the removal of asbestos flooring.
Officials report that building owners adjusted and complied with
the new rules with little complaint. Circumvention of the law is
certainly possible, but those who are caught exposing workers to asbestos—as now there is clear proof the owner knew the dangers—
can be fined heavily and prosecuted for a federal felony.

Even if new asbestos-containing products are banned in the United States, effective abatement laws and greatly increased monitoring of asbestos projects are crucial. Those who knowingly expose workers and future building occupants to asbestos fibers must understand they run a considerable risk of detection and prosecution.

The cost of abatement nationwide may exceed more than $100 billion, which in itself is a convincing reason to ban asbestos now. It makes no sense to put a harmful substance in a structure when it will eventually cost an exorbitant amount just to take it out again. Moreover, the cost of doing the abatement correctly is nowhere near the social and medical costs of doing it incorrectly. The enormous medical expenses generated by hundreds of thousands of future asbestos victims could well break the back of the already tenuous medical health insurance system.

Proper enforcement of abatement laws will occur only if lawmakers take the threat of asbestos seriously. It is likely that not one out of every fifty lawmakers across the country even knows that asbestos is still legal in this country. Even fewer know that the dangers are ongoing, although many are aware that asbestos lawsuits are being filed by the hundreds of thousands. They must come to understand that if asbestos is not banned—and if asbestos abatement is not strictly regulated and monitored—than these lawsuits will continue for decades to come.

The story of asbestos does not have a good ending—yet. That ending can be written if lawmakers can be convinced that asbestos remains a grave danger in this country and abroad and public pressure is applied to make the necessary changes.

A critical element of the Ban Asbestos in America Act calls for the expansion of the definition of asbestos. The six so-called types of

asbestos—chrysotile, tremolite, amosite, crocidolite, anthophyllite, and actinolite—were chosen years ago because they were the
most common types used for commercial products. Today, however, it is clear that other similar minerals also cause serious human
health problems. In Libby, for example, most of the harmful fibers
are not tremolite, but richterite and winchite and other amphiboles that are unregulated, but have proven to be equally deadly. It
is only common sense that the definition of asbestos be enlarged
to include these and any other mineral fibers that harm human
health.

At the top of the priority list should be an immediate investigation of talc, which is used in baby powder, makeup, and other
common products. Talc fibers have been proven toxic through the
tragic deaths of scores of talc miners in upstate New York and other
areas. New York's Jefferson County has a mesothelioma rate that is
among the top ten counties in the country. "It really doesn't matter
what you call it," said Peronard. "If it kills people it ought to be
banned."

Banning asbestos and enforcing abatement laws won't solve all the
problems caused by the "magic mineral." There are still a number
of other issues to be addressed. Among them is the need for new
regulations and agency alignments regarding the dangers of exposure from natural outcroppings of asbestos, such as in El Dorado
Hills, California. The land development now occurring on one of
the nation's largest surface deposits of chrysotile, tremolite, and
other amphiboles is upscale and expansive. Hundreds of millions
of dollars are at stake, but so, too, may be the health of thousands
of people moving into the area, the construction workers doing the
initial excavation, and children attending schools built on or near

the asbestos deposits. Jurisdiction over the health issues involved is divided and subdivided between federal, state, and local agencies. As a result, more energy is often expended in bureaucratic squabbling than in finding a solution to this difficult problem. In California and elsewhere, a clear delineation of governmental hierarchy must be established with a lead agency in charge of all asbestos-related issues, from air and soil monitoring to the permitting of new schools and homes in potentially dangerous areas. As Dr. Alan Whitehouse admonished, "People in California and other places that have environmental exposures to asbestos better understand that this is potentially deadly material. If they don't take it seriously then they are damn fools."

The U.S. Geological Survey recently announced it is embarking on a project that calls for the mapping of asbestiform minerals in many parts of the United States. This is good news, but the announcement came with the caveat that the mapping will include as many areas "as time and budget permit." Why there would be a time limit on the project is a curiosity, but our government should ensure that adequate funding is in place to allow the project to be completed.

Also left unresolved to date is the fact that from 1 million to 25 million American homes may still contain potentially deadly Zonolite insulation made from Libby vermiculite. Efforts by the EPA have been unsuccessful in determining the exact number and location of homes that contain Zonolite, but the government should exhaust all efforts to find them. If that is not possible, then a public notice and education program should be undertaken in those areas where Zonolite was most likely marketed. Home owners should be informed as to how they can identify

whether they have Zonolite in their attics and what to do if they
find it.

For asbestos-disease victims, no issue is more important than medical funding for treatment and potential cures for asbestosis and the
variety of cancers the fibers cause. The problem, of course, is that
few people even in the medical field are aware of the numbers of victims and the extent of the dangers. As a result of that and other factors, asbestos-related diseases are rarely on the radar screen when it
comes to medical and research funding. That must change quickly
if we hope to help the thousands of people who suffer from asbestosis, mesothelioma, and the other asbestos-caused cancers. The
federal government must recognize that, in large part, it was due to
its own lack of vigor in enforcing worker safety and consumer protection laws that asbestos has been able to claim so many victims.
Even without that burden of culpability, Congress must take its
obligation to present and future asbestos victims seriously and begin
to fund large-scale research projects into the treatment and potential cure for asbestos-caused diseases.

Any such project should begin in Libby, where the diseases can
be studied in all their forms and stages. The victims there have already exhibited their overwhelming willingness to cooperate with
medical research teams. The community represents an opportunity
for medical researchers to greatly advance their knowledge about all
phases of asbestos-related diseases. To miss this opportunity would
be a tragedy.

Finally, Libby itself needs the nation's help. Although oblique references are made to it on occasion, the asbestos victims in Libby are,

on the whole, too polite and patriotic to state the obvious. While more than $1 billion in private donations from around the country poured into New York City following the September 11 attacks, the victims in Libby have received no outside help. By the time the asbestos there and in the vermiculite around the country is done killing, it may take as many lives as were lost at the World Trade Center. The medical expense of dealing with the sometimes-lengthy asbestos-related sicknesses in Libby will far outstrip the medical needs of the WTC victims. No one in Libby begrudges the support the nation gave to New York; in fact, many Libby residents sent what money they could. Yet, it is hoped, we will recognize that Libby, too, is a community ravaged by an entity that intentionally sacrificed human lives.

There are those who insist the story of asbestos can be properly seen as the age-old struggle between good and evil. They argue that while profits are important—indeed, they are what make America work— nothing is as important as a human life. But in the end, the story is perhaps reduced simply to a series of images and sounds, moving from the blue asbestos that rained down upon the African Bantu children to the white linen of the lobster lunch with the Browns in New York. It includes the silence of the scar on the mountain above Libby and the voices of lawyers and judges of the bankruptcy court negotiating away the future. Yet the most poignant image of all may be that of the silhouette of the ex–lawman and fighter pilot gazing quietly out the window of his apartment overlooking the baseball field at Libby. The field is empty now, although some high school players will come down to scrimmage later on. Bob Wilkins has on his T-shirt that reads: LOCAL 361 GAVE ME A WATCH, W. R. GRACE GAVE ME ASBESTOS.

A few moments before, he had trouble getting up and walking

across the living room for a glass of water. He has every right to be bitter. He is in pain every day. The damage to his lungs is irreversible. Yet when he was asked how he felt about the company that had contributed to his exposure to the fibers, Wilkins looked out over the ball field and thought for a long time.

"I've tried hard all my life not to have the word 'hate' in my vocabulary," he said finally, in little more than a whisper. "But we were lied to and cheated out of years of our lives. I don't hate them, but I don't have any respect for them, and maybe, in the end, that's the worst thing you can say about a man."